Slim Snacks

More Than 200 Delectable Low-Calorie Snacks That Can Be Made in Minutes

Sharon Sanders

Contemporary Books, Inc.
Chicago

Library of Congress Cataloging in Publication Data

Sanders, Sharon.
  Slim snacks.

  Includes index.
  1. Reducing diets—Recipes.   2. Snack foods.
I. Title.
RM222.2.S24   1982   641.5'635   82-45431
ISBN 0-8092-5781-5

All calorie counts are approximate and are based on figures from the following sources:

Agricultural Handbooks Nos. 8, 8-1, 8-2, and 456, Agricultural Research Service, United States Department of Agriculture.

and

The Barbara Kraus 1981 Revised Edition Calorie Guide to Brand Names and Basic Foods (Signet, New American Library).

Published by Contemporary Books, Inc.
180 North Michigan Avenue, Chicago, Illinois 60601
Manufactured in the United States of America
Library of Congress Catalog Card Number: 82-45431
International Standard Book Number: 0-8092-5781-5

Published simultaneously in Canada by
Beaverbooks, Ltd.
150 Lesmill Road
Don Mills, Ontario M3B 2T5
Canada

To W.C.S.
"Thanks for the inspiration."

Contents

Preface

I am not a diet doctor or a quick-weight-loss snake oil salesman promoting the latest no-fail gimmick diet. I am a cooking teacher and food writer with a great love for good food. *Slim Snacks* evolved as an extension of my basic cooking philosophy: start with the freshest, finest ingredients available and do everything in preparing them to maintain their taste appeal, eye appeal, and nutritional appeal.

Living in Italy for several years and traveling through other European countries, I came to realize how profoundly different the eating habits of the average Italian or Frenchman are when compared with those of the average American. Dining in these European countries is a most pleasurable part of the day, a time that is looked forward to and savored. Even a simple midmorning snack, eaten in the congenial atmosphere of the local café, becomes something of a social event.

Eating in America, for the vast majority, has become a hurry-up affair. In the mad rush for the fastest—and hence most processed—meal, many of us have lost the true pleasure of the taste of good food. The real appetite satisfaction—flavor—that Europeans derive from meals of fresh, unprocessed food is missing in most American processed meals. This lack of flavor may be a major reason why Americans turn to artificially flavored, nutritionally empty, high-calorie snacks. *Slim Snacks* offers habitual nibblers a much-needed alternative to "phony food" snacks—healthful, zesty, appealing, nutritious snacks that are easy to prepare and easy to enjoy.

1

The Slim-Snacks Plan of Attack

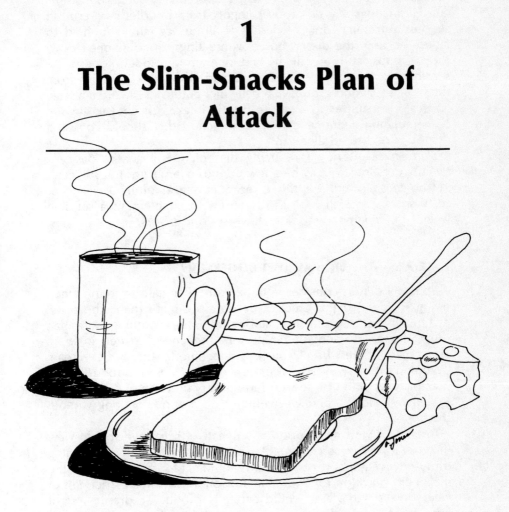

Most gimmick weight loss schemes revolve around banishing one or more types of foods, like starches or fats, from the diet. Dieters are promised that once these villains are banned, weight loss will miraculously occur. This approach is a potentially dangerous shortcut. Eliminating any one food category from the diet can result in serious nutritional deficiencies. It is almost certainly doomed to failure because the dieter, bored with eating from only one or two food groups, is more likely to binge on forbidden foods. The sensible way to lose weight is to include moderate portions from the basic four food groups in a daily diet and to use a kitchen scale and calorie counter to measure caloric intake. Of course, anyone contemplating a dramatic weight reduction diet should consult a doctor or registered dietician.

Slim Snacks is *not* a reducing diet plan. It's for the basically healthy person who may be a few pounds overweight but still can't say no to snacking. For this eater, *Slim Snacks* offers a wealth of zesty snack ideas. It can also be used to supplement a sensible weight-loss regimen with tasty, lower-calorie snacks.

CALORIES—THE BIG BAD DIET BOGEYMAN

So many dieters consider nothing more than calorie counts when trying to lose weight. Calories become the bogeyman—the scary, evil things that make us fat. Calories are, in fact, nothing more than units of measurement that represent the energy stored in food. How many times have you heard someone on a diet moan, "Wouldn't it be wonderful if there were no calories in food?" Well, it actually wouldn't be so wonderful. Every function of our bodies is fueled by calories, and we wouldn't be around for long without them.

Instead of viewing calories as a negative threat, we should view them as a positive challenge. Anyone concerned with maintaining trim body weight and good health should eat foods that contain the maximum nutrition for the minimum calorie count. A strict diet of celery sticks and water would certainly produce a drastic weight loss, but it would also damage good health and sound body function. That is why gimmick diets are so dangerous. By eliminating certain foods from the diet, they also cut essential nutrients.

THE BASIC FOUR

Foods are divided into four basic categories according to their predominant nutrients. One must eat something from each category every day to maintain long-term good health.

The Milk-Cheese Group: These foods supply calcium, riboflavin, protein, vitamin A, and vitamin D (in fortified milk).

The Meat-Poultry-Fish-Beans Group: This group includes meats, poultry, fish, shellfish, nuts, dried beans, peas, lentils, and dried seeds such as sesame and sunflower. These foods provide protein, phosphorus, and iron.

The Vegetable-Fruit Group: These provide vitamin A and vitamin C as well as important dietary fiber.

The Bread-Cereal Group: The foods in this group include bread, packaged cereals, pastas, rice, and whole or cracked grains. They supply thiamine, niacin, riboflavin, and iron. Whole, unprocessed grains and cereals are the most important source of complex carbohydrates in the diet and also provide essential dietary fiber.

Any individual with special dietary problems should consult a registered dietician. A family doctor or local dietician's group can recommend a good one. For those interested in the latest nutritional research, *Jane Brody's Nutrition Book* (Norton) is a valuable reference work. Written in an informative, down-to-earth style, the book presents up-to-date information on many nutrition issues.

THE SLIM-SNACKS CONCEPT

Even the highly respected food scientists who sit on the Food and Nutrition Board of the National Academy of Sciences acknowledge that our present understanding of nutritional needs is incomplete and that the human requirements for many nutrients have not yet been established. *The way to insure good nutrition is to eat a wide variety of fresh foods. Slim Snacks* presents just such a variety of foods for snacking.

These snacks go far beyond what are usually considered snack foods: they include fresh fruits, vegetables, meat and fish dishes, egg preparations, soups, and breads. With such a well-rounded selection of snack foods, *snacks* need no longer be a dirty word to the dieter.

Slim snacks embody three important elements:

- variety
- small portions
- lower-calorie, real-food substitutions for high-calorie foods (for example, substituting low-fat skim-milk yogurt for high-fat mayonnaise in a salad dressing)

Small amounts of high-calorie *real* food flavorings, such as olive oil and maple syrup, are used occasionally because I believe that even small amounts of these genuinely flavorful foods provide more appetite satisfaction than any amount of *phony* flavorings.

Slim Snacks is more than a book of snack recipes. I like to think of it as a source book of delicious ideas for lower-calorie cooking. Many of the condiments and cooking techniques used in *Slim Snacks* should trigger cooking ideas of your own.

HOW TO USE THE RECIPES IN THIS BOOK

Slim Snacks is designed for people who like to eat and like to cook. For those not used to cooking with fresh foods, *Slim Snacks* provides detailed instructions in every recipe. Nothing is left to guesswork. It should come as a very pleasant surprise that cooking from scratch is not the drudgery depicted on TV by the processed-food hucksters. Preparing fresh food can be a very satisfying aspect of everyday life for all members of the family. Cooking with fresh foods gives you the satisfaction of bypassing additive-laden foods and controlling the seasoning of your food.

Whenever possible, recipe measurements are given by weight. For the dieter trying to maintain accurate calorie counts, weighing food portions is the most accurate method. For more information about kitchen scales, turn to page 18.

Most of the snacks are quickly prepared in a matter of minutes; others require a bit more time. Almost all the recipes can and should be included in family meals. Serving suggestions for incorporating the snacks into meals are included throughout the book.

The majority of recipes are for only one or two portions, so the dieter will not be encouraged to oversnack. Most of these, though, can easily be doubled or tripled for use in family meals. The calorie counts given are for relatively small snack portions. If increasing the portions, just multiply the number of snack portions by the calorie count per snack to determine the total calories in the recipe. Divide the total calories by the new number of portions to get the new calorie count per portion.

Many people these days are brown-bagging lunches. Why not save money and increase nutrition by carrying slim snacks to work for both lunch and break-time snacks? It might seem like more of a bother than hitting the nearest vending machine or pastry cart, but the benefits are well worth a little preplanning. Slim snacks are better for you than a pastry or a candy bar, which provide little nutrition and plenty of fat, sugar, salt, and empty calories.

CHOOSING GOOD FOODS FOR GOOD SNACKS

The key to the success of these recipes—particularly the fruit and vegetable recipes—is to select foods that are ripe and fresh. This might sound too obvious to state, but a quick glance at the other carts in the supermarket checkout line may convince you otherwise. Where is the flavor in the wasteland of frozen vegetables and canned fruits? When fresh fruits and vegetables do appear in the carts, all too often they are limp and sad-looking or woefully under-ripe. How do you select the most flavorful fruits and vegetables?

Selecting Vegetables

In the summer, grow as many vegetables as you can in a back-yard plot or in patio or balcony container gardens. If this is impossible, try to shop for seasonally fresh foods at local farmer's markets or produce stands. The vegetables at these markets *usually* come from local farmers and are not shipped the great distances that the supermarket vegetables generally are. It pays to ask, though, because some stands may not buy produce grown in your area.

When buying fresh produce in the supermarket, avoid vegetables prepackaged in cellophane. None of us need to pay a higher price for packaged materials and for the labor involved in that packaging, but the prime reason to avoid these packaged items is that the state of ripeness, or often overripeness, is usually hidden from the consumer's eye and touch.

Use your senses: Feel the vegetable, look at it, and smell it. Choose vegetables that are firm, bright, or glossy-looking. Avoid those with obvious bruise marks or wilted leaves. Before shopping, consult an encyclopedia-type cookbook for guidelines on identifying freshness in individual vegetables. An excellent one, which also contains color photographs of many different kinds of foods, is *The Cook Book* (Crown) by Terence and Caroline Conran.

Learn to buy seasonally as much as possible. Don't expect a tomato purchased in a supermarket in January to taste like a vine-ripened August beauty. Use top-quality canned or home-frozen tomatoes for sauces during the winter and await the thrill of eating truly ripe tomatoes in the summer. You will appreciate the full flavor more.

Use fresh vegetables as soon as possible after purchasing them. They probably have already traveled long distances, and the longer they wait, the more nutrients they lose.

Try new or unfamiliar vegetables when you see them in the market. Variety is important.

Truly fresh vegetables, prepared with a minimum of cooking time, such as by steaming or stir frying, surpass frozen and canned vegetables in taste and texture. Once you are accustomed to well-prepared fresh vegetables, it will be difficult to accept anything less.

Selecting Fruits

Many of the guidelines for vegetables also apply to fruits. Growing some of your own fruit or buying from farmer's markets is usually best. In many areas of the country consumers can pick their own fruit, such as strawberries or apples, at fruit farms and orchards. The advantages are twofold: freshness at a lower price.

Unfortunately, because of the predominant system of shipping fruits thousands of miles to market, most of the fresh fruit we buy was picked long before it could ripen fully. Many fruits arrive at the store rock-hard. There are some steps that can be taken to improve the condition of underripe fruit. Although it may never taste as luscious as a perfectly tree- or vine-ripened fruit, you can intervene where nature was interrupted.

Fruits such as pears, plums, bananas, peaches, and pineapples that are purchased underripe can be ripened at home by placing them in a brown paper bag at room temperature (60–70° F.). Putting a ripe fruit or two in the bag with the unripened fruit will facilitate the process. When the fruit is ripe it should be eaten right away or refrigerated.

Fruit can also be ripened in a clear plastic globe called the Fruit Ripener™, which is available in specialty cookware shops and department stores. For more information write to: Jareen Co., 1130 N. Bundy Dr., Los Angeles, CA 99049.

When selecting fruits, keep in mind when the fruit will be eaten. Don't buy rock-hard pears on Friday if you are planning to serve them on Saturday. If you are lucky enough to find perfectly ripe fruit in the supermarket, take it home and enjoy it right away.

In general, all fruits should be firm but yielding when pressed, without obvious blemishes or rotten spots under the skin. It is wise to familiarize yourself with how individual fruits should look at their best. Consult a reference book like *The Cook Book*.

Try new fruits when you see them in the market. Variety and new flavors keep excitement in low-calorie dining.

THE SLIM-SNACKS LARDER

Keeping the larder stocked with low-calorie condiments is a good idea. If you get into the habit of stocking up on tasty, low-calorie flavorings, your palate and your waistline will benefit. The slim-snacks larder is a combination of low-calorie condiments, nutritious natural foods, and a few high-calorie ingredients.

Larder Staples

- A variety of *whole-grain, stone-ground flours* and *unbleached, enriched white flour.* (Store tightly sealed in a cool, dry spot.)
- A variety of whole-grain cereal and dry vegetable foods such as *cornmeal, oatmeal, bulgur, buckwheat groats, lentils, dried beans* and *imported semolina pastas.* (Store well sealed in a cool, dry spot.)
- *Active dry yeast* without preservatives—available in health food stores and some bulk food stores. I have much better results with this type of yeast than with the supermarket variety. One excellent brand is El Molino. After opening, store the yeast in a covered jar in the refrigerator.
- *Virgin olive oil.* Although this is not a low-calorie food, the flavor

of virgin olive oil (the finest-grade oil obtained from a cold pressing) goes a long way to make food delicious. (Store in a cool, dark spot, but not in the refrigerator.)

- *Polyunsaturated vegetable oil.* Use for stir frying and some baked goods in which a tasteless oil is desirable. (Store in a cool, dry spot.)
- *Chinese sesame oil.* This is one of the most distinctive flavors in the world. Be sure to buy the Chinese oil, which is pressed from roasted sesame seeds and has a complex, intense flavor. The cold-pressed, unroasted variety available in health food stores has almost no taste in comparison with the Chinese oil. (Store in a cool, dark spot.)
- *Soy sauce.* If possible, buy a brand imported from Japan or Hong Kong. The Chinese soy sauce is generally stronger, so less is needed for flavoring. If you are concerned about salt intake, salt-free sauce is available in health food stores.
- *Balsamic vinegar.* An Italian vinegar, it is so mellow that it can dress a salad without the aid of high-calorie oil. By law, this vinegar must be aged in a series of wooden casks for at least 10 years, and some premium labels are aged even longer. Balsamic vinegar can be purchased in specialty food shops or department stores. If it is unavailable in your area, you can order it by mail from Williams-Sonoma. For a catalog, write to Mail Order Department, PO Box 3792, San Francisco, CA 94119.
- *Honey* and *pure maple syrup.* These sweeteners have been used in many of the recipes in this book instead of refined white sugar. Honey and maple syrup do not have fewer calories than refined white sugar nor much more nutrient value (you would have to eat large quantities of honey to get an appreciable nutritional benefit). I have chosen to use small amounts of honey and real maple syrup simply for the flavor. If you are going to expend some valuable calories on nutritionally empty food, you should get some flavor in return.
- *Imported Parmesan cheese.* Although not a low-calorie food, a small amount of the superb flavor of true Parmesan goes a long way in making other foods more enjoyable. Buy it by the wedge at a reputable cheese store. Wrap it loosely in plastic or foil and store in the cheese or vegetable compartment of the refrigerator. For maximum flavor, grate the cheese just before using.

Larder Perishables

- *Fresh herbs* and *whole spices.* I list herbs and spices intentionally with the perishables because, contrary to popular thinking, their flavors don't last forever. Once an herb or spice is crushed or ground, the flavoring oils begin to evaporate. For maximum flavor, grind or crush just before using. More detailed information about fresh herbs and whole spices follows in the next section.
- *Skim milk.*
- Slim-snacks yogurt (see recipe, pages 111–112).
- Homemade chicken stock—essential for soups, sauces, flavoring cooked grains, and delicious as a low-calorie snack in itself (see recipe, pages 88–90).
- *Homemade fish stock* (see recipe, page 91).
- *Fresh lemons, limes,* and *oranges.* No bottled juice or concentrate can ever replace the wonderful zip of fresh citrus juice. An added bonus is the flavor and visual delight of freshly grated zest (the colored rind of a citrus fruit).
- *Mustard.* Two varieties, Dijon and horseradish, are used in these recipes. Many other herb- and spice-flavored mustards are available on the market. (Store opened mustard in the refrigerator.)
- *Unsalted butter.* Nothing can match the flavor of real butter, so small amounts of it are used in *Slim Snacks.* Buy unsalted butter. Salt is a preservative that can mask the off flavor of rancid butter.
- *Yellow onions* and *garlic.* These are two vegetables I am never without. The delicious natural sweetness of onions and the hearty pungency of garlic help pep up many bland foods.
- *Red* and *white dry table wine.* Good-quality jug wines from California, Italy, or France are fine for the *Slim Snacks* recipes. Avoid any wine that has the word *cooking* on the label.

FRESH HERBS ARE THE FINEST

Why use fresh herbs instead of dried? The answer is *flavor.* The taste, texture, and bright color of fresh herbs far surpass those of the dry variety. My cooking students are constantly amazed by the difference fresh herbs make. I am encouraged to see more and more stores—supermarkets, gourmet food shops, and nurseries—

selling fresh herbs. I hope this is one food trend that will continue to grow.

If fresh herbs are impossible to buy in your area, the solution is to grow your own. Most herbs are very easy to grow from seeds and require little care. They can be grown in a garden, in containers, in a pot on a bright windowsill, or under grow lights. Consult your library or agricultural extension service about the best herb gardening techniques for your particular climate. If your local nursery or plant store doesn't carry herb plants or seeds, you can order them by mail from one of the following sources.

J. A. Demonchaux Co., Inc.
827 N. Kansas
Topeka, KS 66608

Nichols Garden Nursery, Inc.
1190 N. Pacific Hwy.
Albany, OR 97321

Le Jardin du Gourmet
West Danville, VT 05873

Home Drying and Freezing

Herbs are aromatic, temperate-climate plants whose seeds or leaves are used to flavor food. When the seeds or leaves are crushed or exposed to heat, their essential flavoring oils are released. Some herbs, if dried properly by the home gardener, can retain good flavor through the winter. Some herbs also freeze well. To dry herbs, cut the branches with the leaves on, brush any superficial dirt from the leaves, and spread them on a screen in a dark, dry place. Or bunch the branches together and tie tightly with string or twine. Tie the bunch from a rafter in a dry, dark spot or from a rod in a cool, dark closet. When the leaves crumble easily to the touch with no hint of moisture left, they are ready to be stored. Place them in a plastic bag and seal tightly or gently remove the leaves from the branches and store in a jar or bag in a cool, dark spot.

To freeze herbs: Remove the leaves from the plant and brush off any superficial dirt. If the leaves are extremely dirty, wash quickly in cold water and dry very well. Place the leaves in plastic bags or containers and seal well. Place in the freezer.

The most advantageous method of preserving each herb is indicated in the following list.

Basil (*Ocimum basilicum*—Annual)
Best preservation method: Freezing
Cooking time: Little or no cooking

This fresh herb heads my list of favorites. Its distinctive mintlike flavor is a highlight of summer cooking, especially when married with garden-ripe tomatoes in salads and sauces. To encourage leaf growth, pinch off the edible flower buds that form at the center of the plant. The buds are more strongly flavored than the leaves, so a smaller amount is required to flavor a dish.

Bay Leaf (*Laurus nobilis*—Perennial)
Best preservation method: Drying or freezing
Cooking time: Responds well to long cooking

An indispensable kitchen herb for marinades, stocks, and stews. The plant is a perennial but must winter indoors in climates with harsh winters. If buying dried bay leaves, always look for whole Turkish bay leaves. Never use ground bay leaf unless you grind it fresh just before cooking.

Chives (*Allium schoenoprasum*—Perennial)
Best preservation method: Freezing (cut before freezing; see following method)
Cooking time: Little or no cooking

This perky herb survives even the harshest winter to add a bright green note to the herb garden very early in the spring. Its mild onion flavor enhances vegetables, salads, eggs, and fish. Always cut chives with a sharp knife or scissors near the root of the plant. To chop chives, bunch some tightly together with one hand. With a sharp knife in the other hand, cut small slices from the bunch. This gives much better flavor and texture than just randomly chopping the chives.

Coriander (*Coriandrum sativum*—Annual)
Best preservation method: Freezing the green leaves and drying the seeds

Cooking time: Green leaves—little or no cooking
Dry seeds—respond to long cooking

The fresh leaves of the coriander plant are often labeled *cilantro* or *Chinese parsley*. They resemble flat-leaf parsley but have a piquant aroma and flavor reminiscent of lemon. Pinch back the flowers to keep the green leaves growing as long as possible. Once the plants go to seed, the seeds can be picked off and dried. To use the seeds, grind or crush as you would whole spices, described later in this chapter.

Dill (*Anethum graveolens*—Annual)
Best preservation method: Freezing the green leaves and drying the seeds
Cooking time: Green leaves—little or no cooking
Dry seeds—respond to long cooking

The unique refreshing flavor of fresh dill leaves is a natural with fish and vegetables. Dried dill seeds can also add spark to breads and vegetables. To use the seeds, grind or crush as you would whole spices.

Fennel (*Foeniculum vulgare*—Perennial)
Best preservation method: Freezing the green leaves and drying the seeds
Cooking time: Green leaves—little or no cooking
Dry seeds—respond to long cooking

Wild or common fennel is the plant that is grown strictly as an herb. But its first cousin, Florence fennel (Foeniculum dulce), can be grown as an herb and a vegetable (see fennel recipe, pages 52–53). Both plants sport foliage that resembles dill. The French and Italians dry the stalks and grill fish over them. The sweet flavor of fennel resembles anise, but I find fennel more delicate. To use the seeds, grind or crush as you would whole spices.

Marjoram (*Marjorana hortensis*—Perennial)
Best preservation method: Drying or freezing
Cooking time: Responds well to fairly long cooking time, especially if dried

The marjoram plant resembles oregano but has smaller, more delicate leaves and small knobs on the tips of the stems. It is sometimes called *knotted marjoram*. Its flavor is a little lighter than oregano and, like oregano, it dries well. In fact, it seems to take on added sweetness when dried.

Mint (*Mentha species*—Perennial)
Best preservation method: Freezing the leaves for fruit salads
Drying the leaves for mint tea
Cooking time: Little or no cooking

There are so many varieties of mint that it would be difficult to list them all. Spearmint and peppermint are two popular varieties that are special in summer cooking, both as flavorings and as delightful edible garnishes for drinks, fruit salads, and desserts. Once it takes hold in the garden, mint is seemingly indestructible. It spreads out runners that quickly take root. If you want to start with a no-fail herb, try mint.

Oregano (*Origanum vulgare*—Perennial)
Best preservation method: Drying or freezing
Cooking time: All forms respond well to fairly long cooking time

For me, oregano always evokes pleasurable memories of robust meals I've enjoyed in Mediterranean countries. Best known for its contribution to pizza, oregano can also flavor soups, omelets, and grilled chicken. It is one Mediterranean perennial that is hardy enough to stand up to nasty northern winters.

Parsley (*Petroselinum crispum*—Biennial)
Best preservation method: Parsley is one herb that is available fresh in all parts of the country year-round; therefore, I would recommend always using it fresh. If you have a large crop in the summer, it can be frozen.
Cooking time: Green leaves—little or no cooking
Stems—respond well to long cooking

Flat-leaf, or Italian parsley, is much more flavorful than the ubiquitous curly variety. Parsley is a much neglected herb, often being used strictly as a garnish. It has a wonderful fresh flavor all its own and can be counted on to add a summer note to foods all year-round. The stems are an essential part of a *bouquet garni*—a combination of parsley, bay leaf, and thyme—which flavors soups, stews, and braised dishes. To make a *bouquet garni,* place the herbs in a small square of cheesecloth. Gather the corners of the cloth at the top and tie tightly with kitchen twine. Drop into the stew or soup. When finished cooking, use a large spoon to press out any juice that may be in the *bouquet garni,* and then discard. If using fresh herbs that are still on the branch, just bind them tightly with several rounds of kitchen twine and drop the bundle into the soup or stew. Before serving, discard the bundle.

Rosemary (*Rosmarinus officinalis*—Perennial)
Best preservation method: Drying or freezing
Cooking time: Responds well to long cooking

Rosemary is a delightful herb plant that looks like a small pine tree. The spiky leaves impart a resinous flavor to foods. Mediterranean cooks waft burning rosemary branches over grilled meats to add a subtle flavor note. Rosemary is a perennial, but its Mediterranean soul cannot endure the winters in much of the United States. Rosemary can be kept inside successfully during the winter under a grow light, then returned outside when the summer sun returns.

Sage (*Salvia officinalis*—Perennial)
Best preservation method: Freezing or drying
Cooking time: Responds well to long cooking

The zesty flavor of fresh sage leaves is far superior to the sometimes sharp taste of the dry leaves. Sage is commonly used with chicken, but it also does wonders with lamb, pork, liver, and some vegetables and breads.

Summer Savory (*Satureia hortensis*—Annual)
Best preservation method: Freezing
Cooking time: Little or no cooking

An annual that is nicknamed the *bean herb* because of its unique affinity with fresh and dried beans. It can also be used with fish, salads, and omelets.

French Tarragon (*Artemisia dracunculus*—Perennial)
Best preservation method: Freezing
Cooking time: Responds best to short cooking

French tarragon produces slender green leaves with a pleasantly mild anise flavor that complements fish, vegetable, and fowl dishes. French tarragon can be propagated only from cuttings, so beware of anyone who tries to sell you "French tarragon seeds." There ain't no such critter. These seeds are from a relative called Russian tarragon, which is virtually tasteless. Tarragon plants should be well mulched to survive harsh northern winters.

Thyme (*Thymus species*—Perennial)
Best preservation method: Freezing or drying
Cooking time: Responds well to long cooking

There are many, many varieties of this seemingly indestructible herb. *T. vulgaris* grows into a small shrub with woody stems and dainty green leaves. *T. serpyllum* creeps along the ground. Most widely used for flavoring soups and stews in a *bouquet garni* (see parsley), thyme can also do wonders for many vegetables and meat dishes.

For more detailed information about growing these and other herbs, *A Cook's Guide to Growing Herbs, Greens and Aromatics* (Alfred A. Knopf) by Millie Owen is an excellent reference book.

THE SPICES OF LIFE

Spices are parts of tropical or subtropical plants used for flavoring food. Unlike herbs, whose leaves or seeds are used for flavoring, spices usually come from other parts of the plants. Some examples are roots, bark, fruits, flower buds, and seed pods. Spices, like herbs, contain essential flavoring oils that begin to evaporate when they are ground. When you buy a preground spice in the supermarket you have no way of knowing how long it has sat in some warehouse. The flavor may be long gone before you even open the can or jar. When spices are kept in their whole state—like a whole nutmeg—they can retain their flavor for years. When buying spices, seek a source that carries whole spices in bulk so that you can purchase small amounts. Look for a store that has a rapid turnover.

Store spices at home in a cool, dark spot and grind just before using, if possible.

Many spices and dried herb seeds can be ground in small electric spice grinders or coffee grinders. A mortar and pestle can also be used. Some, like whole nutmeg, must be grated on the fine side of a vegetable grater or on a small nutmeg grater. Some spices can be used whole, such as cinnamon stick or vanilla bean, to flavor a fruit salad or custard. After using, the whole spice can be rinsed, dried, and used again.

Following is a list of spices used in *Slim Snacks*.

Allspice *(Pimenta dioica)* tastes like a combination of cinnamon, cloves, and nutmeg; hence the name. It is a hard, brown berry that is bigger and smoother than a peppercorn.

Cardamom *(Elettaria cardamomum)* comes in beige, pulpy pods the size of peas. The pods are broken open with a knife or the fingers to release the tiny black seeds inside. These seeds are ground to obtain the distinctive cardamom flavor so widely used in baking.

Cinnamon *(Cinnamomum zeylanicum)* is the dried bark of the cinnamon tree, which is rolled to make cinnamon sticks. The sticks can be used whole or ground to flavor poached fruit, custards, and baked goods.

Cloves *(Eugenia caryophyllus)* look like little brown nails and have a sharp, penetrating flavor to match. Used in combination with the warmer cinnamon and nutmeg, cloves are marvelous in fruit compotes and baked goods.

Fresh gingerroot *(Zingiber officinale)*, with its pungent pepper and citrus flavor, is a trademark of Oriental cooking. If a recipe calls for fresh gingerroot, do not substitute the dried powder. Peeled, fresh gingerroot, covered with dry white wine, will keep in the refrigerator for weeks.

Black peppercorns *(Piper nigrum)* are the dried, not-quite-ripe berries of the pepper vine. They are best if ground, just before using, in a pepper grinder.

Cayenne pepper *(Capsicum frutescens longum)* is made from ground, dried, long red cayenne peppers. You can buy the peppers from a reliable spice merchant and grind them in a spice grinder or buy them already ground from a merchant who keeps a fresh stock on hand.

White peppercorns come from the same plant as the black peppercorns. They are picked after they are ripened, then soaked and rubbed to remove their husks. They are then dried. White pepper isn't as aromatic as the black; it is generally used when the appearance of black specks in the dish would be undesirable.

Paprika (*Capsium frutescens grossum*) is ground from the ripe dried pods of large sweet red peppers. This is one spice that you have to buy preground. Buy an imported Hungarian brand, like Pride of Szeged, for the authentic flavor.

Poppy seeds (*Papaver somniferum*) are delicious blue-black seeds that add texture, color, and flavor interest to breads, salads, and vegetables.

Sesame seeds (*Sesamum indicum*) are used to enhance foods in a variety of cuisines from the Middle East to the Orient. Toasting brings out the rich flavor of the seeds.

Nutmeg (*Myristica fragrans*) has a warm spicy flavor that benefits fresh cheese dishes, fruits, and pastries.

Vanilla bean and pure vanilla extract (*Vanilla planifolia*). The very flowery, rich aroma of a real vanilla bean is somewhat intoxicating. Vanilla beans should be kept tightly wrapped in plastic or in a jar in a cool, dark spot. Pieces of the bean can be used in custards or fruit salads, then dried and used again. If vanilla beans are unavailable, use pure vanilla extract. The artificial extract tastes ghastly.

Salt is actually a mineral, not a spice. The recipes in this book use kosher salt, a pure semicoarse salt with no "free-flowing" additives. If a finer texture is desired, kosher salt can be ground in a spice grinder or mortar and pestle before using.

SLIM SNACKS EQUIPMENT

Spice grinder or **mortar and pestle:** One or the other is necessary for grinding and crushing whole spices and herb seeds. They are both available in specialty kitchenware shops and in cookware sections of department stores. Mortars and pestles come in a variety of materials such as wood, unglazed porcelain, stone, and marble. I prefer stone or porcelain because the slightly rough texture provides friction for easier grinding. Whichever you prefer, check to see that the mortar and pestle are of the same material. If one part is harder than the other, the softer part will wear down too quickly.

Pepper mill or **grinder:** A sturdy wooden mill that is easy to refill is terrific. One very good brand of mill is the Peugeot. For convenience, it is nice to have two mills—one for black pepper and one for white. Pepper can also be ground in a mortar and pestle.

Kitchen scale: Select a model that is sturdy, easy to read, and registers in quarter-ounces, ounces, and pounds, up to five pounds.

Knives: Sharp heavy-duty knives are essential for efficient cooking. Choose knives that are made of a combination of carbon steel (for sharpness) and stainless steel (for easy maintenance). Knives forged from a single piece of steel that runs through the length of the handle are the most durable. A sharpening steel is needed to realign the cutting edge every time you use a knife. Knives also need to be reground periodically, depending on use (every six months is about average). Two knives are essential: a 2- to 3-inch paring knife and a 10- to 12-inch chef's knife. Other good knives to have: a 5- to 6-inch utility knife, a boning knife, and a carving knife.

Food processor or **food mill:** The processor is not essential, but it cuts work time and can contribute a variety of shapes and textures to the diet. Some of the slim snacks, such as the Orange Dream and Delectable Whipped Dairy Topping, are made best in the processor.

When shopping for a processor, look for one you can see demonstrated and that carries a good guarantee. With processors you seem to get what you pay for. The more expensive models are consistently ranked at the top of the consumer test ratings.

If you can't afford a processor and would like to puree sauces and soups quickly, buy a food mill. The food mill is an inexpensive piece of equipment that functions well. It has a rotary plate that forces the food through a sieve disc. Some food mills come with three sieve discs for a variety of puree textures.

Citrus juicer: Juicers range from inexpensive, sturdy plastic models that work quite well to more expensive electric models. One excellent citrus juicer fits onto some food processors.

Citrus zester: Although I generally don't like to clutter my kitchen with gadgets, this is one I couldn't do without. A sturdy plastic handle attached to a piece of V-shaped stainless steel with five sharp holes set into the end makes the zester easy to grasp. When the zester is pulled along the citrus fruit, it removes the zest (the colored part of the rind) in long strips and leaves behind the bitter white pith. The zest can be left in strips or chopped with a knife.

Four-sided vegetable or cheese grater: This tool is good for grating cheeses and vegetables in a variety of consistencies. Citrus zest, gingerroot, and hard cheeses can be grated on the finest side.

Electric mixer or **large balloon whisk:** One or the other is needed for whipping air into egg whites.

Pastry scraper: A flat piece of metal that fits into a tube-shaped handle, the pastry scraper is handy for lifting and cutting doughs and for lifting chopped ingredients into a pan.

Cooking pots and pans: Any heavy, even heat conductor like enameled cast iron or aluminum is suitable for these recipes. Some of the recipes specify nonaluminum pans for cooking acidic foods like tomatoes, or green vegetables like spinach, because these foods will react chemically with the aluminum and will discolor during cooking. A 12-quart stockpot is necessary for the Homemade Chicken Stock. A rolled-steel wok is good to have for the stir frying recipes, but a 12-inch heavy skillet will also work well.

Baking pans: Some of the recipes require nonstick baking pans: an 8-inch square pan, several large baking sheets, a 10-inch tube pan, and one or two 8½″ × 4½″ × 2½″ bread pans.

Baking stone: A baking stone is a ceramic rectangle or circle fired at a very high temperature. When bread is baked on a preheated baking stone it develops a crisp crust and extra light texture characteristic of bread baked in an old-fashioned brick oven. For more information about baking stones, see Chapter 6.

Instant-reading thermometer: A small glass temperature dial that sits atop a metal rod, an instant-reading thermometer is a convenient tool to check food temperatures such as roasts, the yeast water for bread baking, and delicate custard sauces that must not boil.

Steamer rack: An inexpensive adjustable rack made of stainless steel or a more expensive bamboo steamer may be used. It is important to have a pan deep enough to comfortably hold the steamer rack and food to be steamed so that they can be covered with the pot lid.

Small spoon-whisk: A small spoon-shaped tool with a coil on the end is useful for emulsifying small amounts of salad dressing.

2
Virtuous Vegetable Snacks

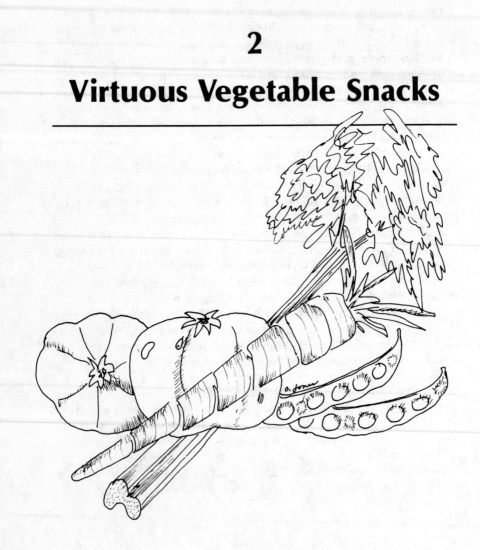

Vegetables are the dieter's best friend. Low in fat and high in nutrients and natural fiber, vegetables supply a tremendous amount of variety and flavor in the diet.

The shapes and colors of mounds of fresh vegetables at a farmer's market can provide real inspiration to the cook. Cooking techniques such as broiling, stir frying, steaming, and baking, combined with a cornucopia of fresh herbs and freshly ground spices, turn these inspirations into delicious reality.

These vegetable snacks are too good to eat only at snack time. Serve them at mealtime as tasty first courses, vegetable side dishes, and salads. Hopefully, this chapter will acquaint you with some unfamiliar vegetables, which you and your family will enjoy for years to come.

Many of the recipes in this chapter are equally delicious eaten hot, at room temperature, or slightly chilled. Many of these vegetable dishes benefit from not being chilled at all, but if the snack must be prepared in advance and refrigerated, try to remove it about 10–15 minutes before eating. If a food is too cold, the flavor will be masked. Salads composed of delicate greens are always best when dressed at the last minute to maintain crispness. If making a salad to take to work as a snack, simply pack the dressing separately and toss just before eating.

For the crunchaholics among you, I hope that you reach for a vegetable snack instead of a bag of crunchy "nothing food." The texture, color, and flavor are much more satisfying.

VEGETABLE SALADS

Shredded Carrots in Cucumber Rounds

This snack makes an excellent, colorful, low-calorie party hors d'oeuvre.

Preparation time: about 10 minutes
Portions: 15
Calories per portion: 11

1 14-ounce seedless English
   cucumber
3 ounces carrot, trimmed of
   stem end
¼ ounce chives or green part
   of scallion

2 teaspoons virgin olive oil
1 teaspoon white wine vinegar
⅛ teaspoon kosher salt
2 grinds black pepper

Scrub the cucumber and trim the ends. Cut into 15 ½-inch rounds. With a melon baller or small spoon, scoop out the center of each round, taking care not to scoop all the way through. Discard the scooped-out portions and set the cucumber rounds aside.

Scrub the carrot, then shred on the coarse side of a vegetable grater. If using chives, bunch them tightly together with one hand and slice thinly with a sharp knife. If using scallion green, chop fine.

Mix the carrots and chives. Season with oil, vinegar, salt, and pepper. Toss to combine. Spoon the shredded carrots into the cucumber rounds. Chill, if desired, before eating.

Stuffed Cherry Tomatoes

These tasty tomatoes are stuffed with Neufchâtel, a cheese almost identical to cream cheese in texture and flavor but which has about 25 percent fewer calories.

Preparation time: 10 minutes
Portions: 13
Calories per portion: 15

13 cherry tomatoes, weighing 9
   ounces
2 ounces Neufchâtel cheese at
   room temperature

2 teaspoons apple juice
1 teaspoon fresh basil or mint
Freshly ground black pepper

Cut the tops from the tomatoes. Over a small dish gently squeeze the sides of the tomatoes together to remove the seeds. Set the tomatoes on a plate.

Cream the cheese until it is very smooth, gradually adding the apple juice. Cream well. If using basil leaves, roll them into a tight bundle, then slice thin. If using mint, chop very fine. Mix with the cheese. Add 1–2 grinds of black pepper and mix. With a small spoon, stuff the tomatoes with the cheese mixture. These tomatoes can be made in advance and refrigerated for 1–2 days.

Triple-Tasty Bean Salad

This three-bean salad, made with fresh green and yellow beans and dried kidney beans, has far better flavor and texture than the sweetened deli variety made from mushy canned beans.

Preparation time: about 45 minutes (with beans already soaked)
Portions: 6
Calories per portion: 74

**2 ounces dried red kidney
  beans**
½ ounce yellow onion
½ ounce celery
**½ ounce carrot, trimmed of
  stem end**

8 ounces yellow snap beans
8 ounces green beans
1 ounce yellow onion
**1 tablespoon summer savory or
  Italian parsley**

DRESSING

1 tablespoon virgin olive oil
**2 tablespoons balsamic vinegar
  or high-quality aged red
  wine vinegar**

¼ teaspoon kosher salt
4–5 grinds black pepper

Place the kidney beans in a small bowl and cover with water. Set aside to soak for 12 hours.

Drain the kidney beans and rinse. Place them in a small saucepan and cover with cold water. Coarsely chop ½ ounce each of onion, celery, and carrot and add to the pan. Cover and bring the water to a boil over high heat. Reduce the heat to a simmer and cook, partially covered, until the beans are tender but still firm (about 35 minutes). If at any time the water level goes below the beans, add more water to just cover the beans. For the last 5 minutes of cooking, remove the lid and turn the heat up to a rapid simmer. Cook off the liquid, tossing the beans often so as not to burn them. Remove the vegetables and discard. Cool the beans. (This step of soaking and cooking the kidney beans can be done in advance. The cooked beans can be covered and refrigerated for several days.)

Place about 2 inches of water in a 6-quart saucepan. Cover the pan and place over high heat. Wash the yellow and green beans and remove the ends (also remove the strings, if necessary). Set a steamer rack over the water when it comes to the boil and place the beans on the rack. Cover the pan and reduce the heat slightly. Steam the beans until tender but still firm (about 7 minutes). Remove from the steamer and rinse under cold water. Spread on a towel to cool and dry.

Chop 1 ounce of onion very fine. Set aside. Chop the savory very fine and set aside. In a salad bowl, mix together all the dressing ingredients. Cut the green and yellow beans into diagonal pieces. Combine in the salad bowl with the kidney beans, the chopped savory, and the onion. Toss to combine. Eat right away or refrigerate. If refrigerated, let the salad sit at room temperature about 15 minutes before eating.

Mushrooms and Pearl Onions in Thyme Vinaigrette

This snack is a delicious, light dinner appetizer.

Preparation time: about 10 minutes
Marinating time: several hours
Portions: 4
Calories per portion: 42

**8 ounces small button
  mushrooms
7 ounces pearl onions**

MARINADE

1 teaspoon virgin olive oil
1 tablespoon balsamic vinegar
or high-quality aged red
wine vinegar

Pinch of kosher salt
1 teaspoon fresh or frozen
thyme leaves

Fill a 3-quart saucepan with water. Cover and place over high heat.

Clean the mushrooms with a damp mushroom brush or a damp cloth. Cut off the ends of the stems and discard. (If small mushrooms are unavailable, use large ones and cut into quarters or halves to match the size of the onions.)

When the water boils, place the pearl onions in the water. Cover and return to the boil. With a slotted spoon or skimmer, lift the onions from the water into a bowl. Fill the bowl with cold water. Pour out all but 2 inches of the hot water from the saucepan. Cover the pan and set on the stove over low heat.

Skin the onions and cut a small cross into the root of each one. Place an adjustable nonaluminum steamer rack into the saucepan with the hot water. Place the onions on the steamer rack, cover the pan, and steam for 5 minutes. Place the mushrooms on top of the onions and steam 3 minutes more. Transfer the onions and mushrooms to a bowl.

Combine the oil, vinegar, and salt. Chop the thyme and add to the marinade. Toss with the vegetables. Marinate at room temperature, tossing occasionally for 30 minutes. Cover and refrigerate for several hours. Allow to come to room temperature and toss just before eating.

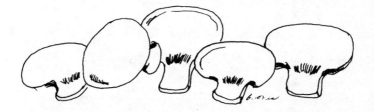

Minted Cucumbers

This is a refreshing summer salad or snack.

Preparation time: about 5 minutes
Soaking time: 30 minutes
Portions: 2
Calories per portion: 36

10 ounces cucumber
½ teaspoon kosher salt
2 ice cubes

DRESSING

1 teaspoon virgin olive oil   **1 teaspoon fresh mint**
2 teaspoons lemon juice   **Freshly ground black pepper**

Scrub the cucumber and trim the ends. Cut in half lengthwise and scoop out the seeds with a sharp spoon or melon baller. Discard the seeds and slice the cucumbers into ¼-inch-thick half-moons. Cover with cold water and the salt. Place the ice cubes in the water and set the cucumbers aside for 30 minutes.

Drain the cucumbers and rinse well with cold water. Drain well and pat dry. Mix the olive oil and lemon juice. Toss with the cucumbers. Chop the mint leaves and add to the salad. Sprinkle with freshly ground black pepper and toss. If the snack is refrigerated, let it sit at room temperature 15 minutes before eating.

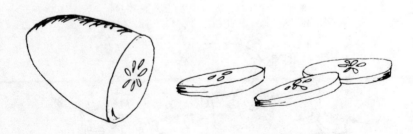

Fresh Tomato and Pepper Relish

This relish is a tangy accompaniment to almost any kind of sand-wich.

Preparation time: about 10 minutes
Marinating time: several hours
Portions: 8
Calories per portion: 42

10 ounces cucumber
7 ounces ripe tomato
7 ounces green or red pepper
6 ounces scallion, white and
    green part, root end
    trimmed

6 ounces celery
1 teaspoon fresh basil, Italian
    parsley, or cilantro

DRESSING

1 tablespoon virgin olive oil
1 tablespoon lemon juice

¼ teaspoon kosher salt
Freshly ground black pepper

Scrub the vegetables and pat dry. Trim the ends from the cu-cumber and slice in half lengthwise. Remove the seeds with a sharp spoon and discard. Cut each half into lengthwise halves and then chop into ¼-inch pieces. Place the cucumbers in a bowl.

Core and halve the tomato. Squeeze gently to press out the seeds. Discard the seeds and cut the tomato into small chunks.

Remove stem and seeds from pepper. Cut into ¼-inch pieces. Add pepper to the other vegetables.

Slice the scallion and add to the other vegetables. Cut the celery rib into lengthwise quarters, then into small chunks. Add to the vegetable bowl.

Chop the herb very fine and sprinkle over the vegetables.

Combine the dressing ingredients and toss with the vegetables. Cover and refrigerate for several hours, tossing occasionally. Allow to come to room temperature before eating. The relish can be refrigerated for up to a week.

Shredded Romaine and Carrot Salad

Instead of always using boring iceberg lettuce for salads, experiment with tastier greens like romaine.

Preparation time: about 3 minutes
Portions: 1
Calories per portion: 22

¾ ounce romaine leaves, with tough center spine removed
1 ounce carrot, trimmed of stem end

1 teaspoon balsamic vinegar or high-quality aged red wine vinegar
Pinch of kosher salt
Freshly ground black pepper

Wash the romaine leaves and pat dry. Lay the leaves on top of one another and roll into a tight bundle. Cut into thin slices with a sharp knife. Unravel and place in a salad bowl.

Scrub the carrot. Shred on the coarse side of a vegetable grater. Place in the bowl with the romaine. Dress with the vinegar, salt, and 2 grinds of black pepper. Toss to coat.

Oriental Mushroom Salad

Preparation time: about 10 minutes
Portions: 4
Calories per portion: 54

8 ounces firm white mushrooms
2 ounces Fresh Bean Sprouts (see Index)

1 ounce scallions, white and green part, root end trimmed

DRESSING

1 teaspoon Chinese sesame oil
2 teaspoons vegetable oil

1 teaspoon imported soy sauce
2 teaspoons white wine vinegar

Clean the mushrooms with a damp mushroom brush or damp cloth. Trim the ends and discard. Slice the mushrooms into ⅛-inch slices. Place them in a bowl along with the bean sprouts. Slice the scallion into inch-long julienne strips. Place in the bowl.

Mix dressing ingredients with a small spoon-whisk until smooth. Pour over the vegetables and toss to coat thoroughly.

Creamy Cucumber Salad

Preparation time: about 5 minutes
Soaking time: 30 minutes
Portions: 2
Calories per portion: 22

8 ounces cucumber
½ teaspoon kosher salt
2 ice cubes

DRESSING

3 tablespoons Slim Snacks Yogurt (see Index)
1 teaspoon balsamic vinegar or high-quality aged red wine vinegar

1 tablespoon fresh or frozen chives
4 grinds of black pepper

Scrub the cucumber and trim the ends. Slice in half lengthwise and scoop out the seeds with a melon baller or spoon. Discard seeds. Slice into ¼-inch half-moons and place in a bowl. Sprinkle with salt and cover with cold water. Place the ice cubes in the bowl. Set the cucumbers aside to soak for 30 minutes.

Mix the yogurt in a bowl with the vinegar. Hold the chives tightly together with one hand and slice thin with a sharp knife. Mix with the yogurt and vinegar and set aside.

Drain the cucumbers and rinse several times with cold water. Drain and pat dry. Put in the bowl with the dressing and toss to coat the cucumbers. Grind black pepper over the top and eat right away or refrigerate.

Broccoli Radish Circular Salad

Preparation time: about 5 minutes
Portions: 1
Calories per portion: 59

3 ounces broccoli stem   **½ teaspoon lemon juice**
2½ ounces radishes   **Freshly ground black pepper**
½ teaspoon virgin olive oil

Place 1 inch of water in a small nonaluminum saucepan. Cover and set over high heat.

Wash the broccoli and radishes. Trim the broccoli end and peel the stem. Cut into circles ⅛ inch thick. When the water boils, place the broccoli circles in the pan. Steam, covered, for 1 minute. Drain and rinse under cold water. (The cooking water can be saved for soup.) Pat the broccoli dry and place in a small bowl.

Trim both ends of the radishes and slice into ⅛-inch-thick circles. Place in the bowl with the broccoli.

Toss with the olive oil, lemon juice, and a grind of black pepper. Eat right away or refrigerate. If refrigerated, let the salad sit at room temperature 15 minutes before eating.

Cauliflower Antipasto

This Cauliflower Antipasto, with its touch of red pepper and garlic, is a fine first course or hors d'oeuvre.

Preparation time: about 10 minutes
Marinating time: 24 hours
Portions: 4
Calories per portion: 30

12 ounces cauliflower flowerets

MARINADE

1 tablespoon virgin olive oil
1 large clove garlic

2 tablespoons balsamic vinegar
or high-quality aged red
wine vinegar
⅛ teaspoon red pepper flakes

Choose a saucepan that is at least 4–5 inches deep and 8–10 inches wide. Fill the pan with 1–2 inches of water. Cover and set over high heat.

Wash the cauliflower. Cut the flowerets into equal-sized pieces. When the water boils, place a nonaluminum adjustable steamer rack into the pan. Reduce the heat so the water is cooking at a brisk simmer. Lay the cauliflower pieces on the steamer rack in a single layer and cover the pan. Steam until the cauliflower is tender but still firm (about 7 minutes).

While the cauliflower is steaming, heat the oil in a small pan. Crush the garlic clove with a heavy knife. Lift off the skin and discard. Put the garlic clove in the pan with the oil. Cook over low heat until the garlic clove starts to brown. Cool slightly, then add the vinegar and hot pepper flakes. Toss with the cooked cauliflower and cool. Cover and marinate in the refrigerator, tossing the mixture several times, for 24 hours. Bring the antipasto to room temperature, drain off the marinade, and discard the garlic clove before eating.

Tomato and Basil Salad

Tomato and fresh basil is a classic combination in Italian cooking. Make this snack with only garden-ripened tomato and fresh basil leaves and you will experience one of the great flavor duets of all time.

Preparation time: about 1 minute
Portions: 1
Calories per portion: 47

7 ounces tomato

2-3 small basil leaves or 1 large leaf

½ teaspoon balsamic vinegar or high-quality aged red wine vinegar

Dash of kosher salt

2 grinds of fresh black pepper

Core the tomato and slice thin. Fan the slices out onto a plate. Place the basil leaves on top of one another and roll into a tight tube. Cut into thin slices and sprinkle over the tomatoes. Sprinkle with vinegar, salt, and pepper. Eat right away.

Green Bean Salad with Mustard Dressing

Preparation time: about 10 minutes
Portions: 2
Calories per portion: 40

5½ ounces young, tender green beans

DRESSING

1 teaspoon virgin olive oil
1 teaspoon horseradish mustard
Pinch of kosher salt

Fill a deep 2-quart saucepan with about 2 inches of water. Cover and place over high heat.

Wash the beans. Remove the ends and discard. When the water comes to the boil, place an adjustable steamer rack in the pan. Lay the beans on the rack and cover the pan. Reduce the heat so the water is at a brisk simmer. Steam the beans until they are tender but still very crisp (about 4 minutes). Remove the beans and rinse under cold running water. Spread on a towel to dry. Save the steaming water for soup.

In a small bowl combine the oil, mustard, and salt with a small spoon-whisk. Add the beans to the bowl and toss to coat with the dressing. Refrigerate, if desired, but let the beans come to room temperature before eating.

Roasted Red Pepper with Balsamic Vinegar

Roasting brings out the natural sweetness in ripe red peppers. This snack is very good served as a first course at a summer dinner.

Preparation time: about 45 minutes
Portions: 1
Calories per portion: 26

1 4-ounce red pepper	**Dash of kosher salt**
½ teaspoon balsamic vinegar or high-quality aged red wine vinegar	**Freshly ground black pepper**

Wash and dry the pepper. Place it 6 inches under an oven broiler or over very hot coals on a barbecue grill. The pepper can be roasted over just-lit charcoal that is flaming and not yet ready to cook other foods or held over a gas burner with a fork. Watch the pepper carefully and turn it when the skin is charred black on the side closest to the heat source. Keep turning the pepper until it is completely charred on all sides. Remove from the heat and place in a plastic bag. Close the bag tightly for 10 minutes.

Remove the pepper from the bag. Using your hands and a small knife, pull the stem and seeds away from the pepper, then remove the skin. Work over the serving dish to preserve the pepper juice. Cut the pepper into thin strips, place on the serving dish, and sprinkle with the vinegar, salt, and pepper. This snack can be refrigerated, but allow it to come to room temperature before eating.

Tarragon Potato Salad

Tarragon Potato Salad is a satisfying yet light addition to summer picnics or *al fresco* dinners.

Preparation time: about 45 minutes
Portions: 8
Calories per portion: 76

1 pound small red potatoes
1 teaspoon kosher salt
1 large egg
1 ounce red onion

1 tablespoon fresh tarragon
leaves or fresh basil, dill, or
cilantro

DRESSING

2 ounces Neufchâtel cheese at
room temperature
2 tablespoons skim milk

2 teaspoons horseradish
mustard or Dijon mustard

Place a small, covered pan of water on the stove to heat.

Meanwhile, scrub the potatoes and cut lengthwise into quarters. Cut each quarter into 4 pieces. Place the cut potatoes in a saucepan and cover with cold water and 1 teaspoon kosher salt. Place over high heat, cover, and bring to a boil. Uncover and simmer until the potatoes are cooked (about 15 minutes). Drain and rinse under cold water. Spread on a towel to cool and dry (about 15 minutes).

When the small pan of water comes to a boil, gently drop the egg into the water and cook, uncovered, at a gentle simmer for 10 minutes. Remove the egg and place in a bowl of cold water for 10 minutes. Remove the egg shell. Set the egg aside to cool for a few minutes more, then chop into small pieces.

Chop the onion very fine. Chop the tarragon leaves very fine.

To make the dressing, in a large bowl blend the Neufchâtel cheese until smooth. Gradually add the milk, using a small spoon-whisk, until the mixture is smooth. Add the mustard and mix.

Place the potatoes, onion, tarragon, and chopped egg in the bowl. Toss gently to coat. Taste and add a sprinkling of salt if desired. The potato salad can be eaten right away or refrigerated for several days.

Tangy, Creamy Coleslaw

Preparation time: about 20 minutes
Portions: 16
Calories per portion: 26

2-pound head of cabbage
4 ounces yellow onion
4 ounces carrot, trimmed of
   stem end

2 ounces celery
1 ounce green banana pepper
   or green bell pepper

DRESSING

1½ cups Slim Snacks Yogurt
   (see Index)

3 tablespoons balsamic vinegar
   or high-quality aged wine
   vinegar
1½ teaspoons kosher salt

Wash the cabbage and remove any discolored outer leaves. Cut into quarters and remove the hard core. Discard. Shred the cabbage on the coarse side of a vegetable grater, slice thin on a vegetable slicer, or slice in the food processor with the slicing disc. Place the shredded cabbage in a bowl and set aside.

Chop the onion very fine. Scrub the carrot and celery. Chop both very fine. Wash the pepper, remove the top, and slice in half lengthwise. Remove the seeds and ribs and discard. Chop very fine. Add the chopped vegetables to the cabbage and toss to combine.

To make the dressing and assemble the coleslaw, in a small bowl mix the dressing ingredients to combine. Pour over the cabbage and toss to coat the cabbage evenly. The coleslaw can be eaten right away or refrigerated for several days.

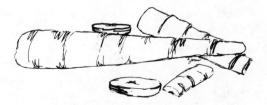

Soy and Sesame Spinach Salad

Preparation time: about 3 minutes
Portions: 1
Calories per portion: 33

**2 ounces spinach leaves,
    trimmed of stems and
    spines**
¼ ounce red onion

DRESSING

¼ teaspoon Chinese sesame oil   **½ tablespoon white wine**
¼ teaspoon imported soy sauce   **vinegar**

GARNISH

¼ teaspoon sesame seeds

Wash and dry the spinach leaves. Tear the leaves into small pieces and place in a bowl. Chop the red onion into small pieces and place in the bowl with the spinach.

Combine the dressing ingredients with a small spoon-whisk. Set aside.

Place the sesame seeds in a small heavy skillet. Over medium-high heat toast the seeds, tossing occasionally, until they are golden brown. Remove from the heat. Toss the dressing with the spinach and onions to coat thoroughly. Garnish with the toasted sesame seeds.

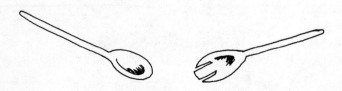

Pickled Beets

These Pickled Beets keep well and make a great relish dish for picnics and summer barbecues.

Preparation time: about 1 hour
Marinating time: 24 hours
Portions: 4
Calories per portion: 53

1 pound fresh beets without tops or 2 pounds beets with green tops
3 ounces red onion
2 tablespoons balsamic vinegar or high-quality aged red wine vinegar

1 bay leaf
2 cloves
3 black peppercorns
¼ teaspoon kosher salt

If using beets with tops, remove the tops and reserve for another use, such as Beet Greens with Lemon (see Index). Cut the beet stems from the beets about 1 inch above the beet. Scrub the beets in cold water and rinse well. Place in a 1½-quart saucepan and cover with cold water. Cover the pan and place on the stove to heat. When the water comes to the boil, remove the lid and reduce the heat to a steady simmer. Cook the beets, skimming foam from the top as it appears, for about 45–50 minutes. The beets are cooked when they are easily pierced with a sharp knife.

While the beets are cooking, peel the onion and slice thin. Set aside.

When the beets are cooked, remove them with a slotted spoon. Place in a colander and run cold water over them.

Add all the remaining ingredients and the sliced onion to the beet water and cook at a rapid simmer until about 1 cup of liquid is left.

Peel the beets by holding them under running cold water and rubbing away the skin. Slice the beets thin. When the beet liquid is reduced to 1 cup, add the sliced beets to the pan and remove from the heat. Allow to cool to room temperature, then refrigerate for at least 24 hours before eating.

The beets will keep, refrigerated, for several weeks. To eat the beets, remove with a slotted spoon. Save the liquid for Pickled Eggs (see Index).

Belgian Endive and Beet Salad

Belgian endive, which resembles a small ear of corn in shape, is a relative of chicory and curly endive. It is available during the winter months. Its pale green and white leaves and pleasantly bitter taste contrast wonderfully with the deep ruby color and sweet flavor of fresh cooked beets.

Preparation time: about 3 minutes, with beets already cooked
Portions: 2
Calories per portion: 37

6½ ounces Belgian endive
4 ounces cooked beets (see
    cooking method for
    Pickled Beets)

DRESSING

2 teaspoons Slim Snacks Yogurt   **1 teaspoon white wine vinegar**
    (see Index)   **Freshly ground black pepper**

Rinse the endive quickly under cold water and pat dry. Cut off the root end. Slice the endive into ¼-inch circles. Arrange the circles on two salad plates. Cut the beet into ¼-inch circles, then into ¼-inch wide sticks. Arrange on top of the endive.

Mix the yogurt and vinegar. Pour over the salad. Garnish with freshly ground black pepper.

Soy Marinated Scallions

Preparation time: about 5 minutes
Marinating time: 24 hours
Portions: 8
Calories per portion: 7

3½ ounces scallions (about 8   **and about ¼ of the green**
    scallions trimmed of roots   **tops)**

MARINADE

1½ teaspoons fresh gingerroot   **½ teaspoon Chinese sesame oil**
1 small clove garlic   **1 teaspoon white wine vinegar**
1 teaspoon imported soy sauce

Select a pan that is at least 8 inches wide and 4–5 inches deep. Fill the pan with 2 inches of water, cover, and set over high heat.

Wash the scallions and slit each one through the center, starting at the green end and running halfway through the white end. When the water comes to the boil, place a nonaluminum adjustable steamer rack in the pan and lay the scallions in a single layer on the steamer. Cover and steam for 1 minute. Remove the scallions and place them in a shallow dish in which they fit tightly.

Chop the gingerroot and garlic very fine. Mix with the other marinade ingredients and pour over the scallions. Cover the dish with plastic wrap and refrigerate for 24 hours. Turn the scallions several times during the marinating period. To serve, remove from the marinade and brush off the garlic and ginger.

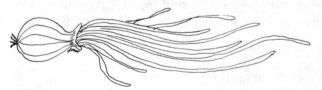

Avocado Mold

Served with the optional tomato and cilantro garnish, this avocado mold makes a refreshing and pretty first course for a dinner party.

Preparation time: about 15 minutes
Chilling time: at least 3 hours
Portions: 10
Calories per portion: 83

1 envelope unflavored gelatin   **4 ounces low-fat cottage**
¾ cup hot water   **   cheese**
¼ cup cold water   **1 pound very ripe avocados**
3 tablespoons lime juice   **½ teaspoon kosher salt**
1 teaspoon grated yellow onion   **Dash of cayenne pepper**

Set a small pan filled with ¾ cup of water over high heat. In a small heatproof cup sprinkle the gelatin over ¼ cup cold water. Place the gelatin cup in the pan with the hot water, double boiler style. Remove from the heat and set aside until the gelatin melts.

Squeeze the lime juice and grate the onion. Place in a blender or in the bowl of a food processor fitted with the steel blade. Add the cottage cheese to the work bowl and process until smooth and creamy.

Cut the avocados in half lengthwise. Lift the seeds out by spearing them with a knife. Discard the seeds. With a spoon, scoop out the avocado flesh, scraping the shell to remove all of it, and place it in the food processor. Process until very smooth, scraping down the sides of the bowl as necessary.

When the gelatin has melted (it will look clear), pour it into the hot water in the pan. Mix well to combine. Mix the salt and cayenne with the gelatin water. With the food processor running, add the gelatin water through the feed tube. Process until it is combined with the avocado mixture. Pour into a 3-cup dish. Cover and chill in the refrigerator until set (at least 3 hours or as long as 24). For a party, the mixture can be poured into a lightly oiled 3-cup mold, then chilled and unmolded (see technique used for Gazpacho Aspic).

TOMATO AND CILANTRO
GARNISH (OPTIONAL)

Calories per portion with garnish: 88

10 ounces ripe tomato
1 tablespoon fresh cilantro
leaves

Halve the tomato. Squeeze each half gently to remove the seeds. Remove the core and discard with the seeds. Chop the tomato into small pieces.

Chop the cilantro fine.

To serve as a first course: Scoop out the avocado mold or unmold and slice into 10 servings. Lay each serving on a lettuce leaf and garnish with the chopped tomato. Sprinkle each serving with the chopped cilantro.

Gazpacho Aspic

This cool tomato aspic with the textural contrast of crisp raw vegetables makes a great do-ahead addition to a large buffet dinner party.

Preparation time: about 10 minutes
Chilling time: at least 4 hours
Portions: 6
Calories per portion: 27

1 envelope unflavored gelatin
¼ cup cold water
2 cups tomato juice
1½ ounces celery
1½ ounces scallion, white and green part, trimmed of root end

1½ ounces green pepper, trimmed of top, ribs, and seeds
4 drops Tabasco sauce or more to taste
⅛ teaspoon kosher salt

GARNISH

Several sprigs of parsley
Lemon slices

Heat a small amount of water in a small covered saucepan. Sprinkle the gelatin over ¼ cup water in a small heatproof cup. Place the cup in the hot water, double boiler style, and turn off the heat. Let the cup sit in the hot water until the gelatin is melted (about 5 minutes).

Heat the tomato juice. Wash and chop the vegetables medium-fine. Combine the melted gelatin with the tomato juice. Add the Tabasco and salt. Add the chopped vegetables. Pour into a 3-cup glass dish. Cover and chill for several hours or overnight, until well set. Scoop out with a large spoon to serve.

To serve the gazpacho as a molded aspic for a party buffet, pour the tomato mixture into a very lightly oiled 3-cup mold. Chill until solid. To unmold, remove from the refrigerator and dip the mold up to the rim in a pan of hot, not boiling, water. Loosen the edges of the aspic with a wet knife or spatula. Rinse the serving plate with cold water and shake off the excess. Place the serving plate on top of the mold and, grasping both dishes firmly in both hands, invert the mold. Lift the mold away from the dish and garnish the aspic.

VEGETABLE STIR-FRIES

Stir frying, a Chinese cooking technique, is a marvelous way to lock texture, flavor, and color into fresh vegetables.

Carrot and Pea Pod Stir-Fry

Preparation time: about 5 minutes
Portions: 2
Calories per portion: 59

SAUCE

¼ teaspoon cornstarch
1 tablespoon Homemade
    Chicken Stock (see Index)
½ teaspoon imported soy sauce

---

2 ounces carrot, trimmed of
    stem end
2½ ounces Chinese pea pods
⅓ ounce scallion, white and
    green part, trimmed of
    root end

1 teaspoon vegetable oil
½ ounce Fresh Bean Sprouts
    (see Index)

Prepare the sauce by dissolving the cornstarch in 1 teaspoon of the chicken stock. Add the remaining stock and the soy sauce. Mix and set aside.

Fill a 1-quart pan with water, cover, and set over high heat.

Scrub the carrot, then cut it into oval-shaped diagonal slices about ¼ inch thick. When the water boils, add the carrots to the water and boil for 1 minute. Drain and rinse with cold water. Pat the carrots dry and set aside.

Wash the pea pods and scallion. Trim the pea pods by grabbing the tufted end and pulling down along the straight side of the pod to remove the string. Cut the pea pods into diagonal pieces about ½ inch wide. Cut the scallion into 1-inch pieces and then into julienne strips. Set aside, keeping the vegetables separate.

Place the vegetable oil in a wok or a heavy 10-inch skillet with sloping sides. Heat the oil until hot but not smoking. Over high heat, toss the carrots in the oil, using Chinese stir-frying utensils or two large spoons. Toss for 1 minute. Add the pea pods and toss for 1 minute more. Remove the pan from the heat and add the scallions and bean sprouts. Pour the sauce over the vegetables and toss for 30 seconds or until the sauce has coated the vegetables. Eat right away.

Broccoli and Celery Stir-Fry

Preparation time: about 5 minutes
Portions: 2
Calories per portion: 51

SAUCE

¼ teaspoon cornstarch
½ tablespoon dry sherry

½ tablespoon Homemade
    Chicken Stock (see Index)
½ teaspoon imported soy sauce

---

3 ounces broccoli flowerets
2 ounces celery
1 teaspoon vegetable oil
1 small clove garlic

1 quarter-sized slice fresh
    gingerroot
½ ounce Fresh Bean Sprouts
    (see Index)

Dissolve the cornstarch in the sherry. Add the chicken stock and soy sauce. Mix and set aside.

Put about 1 inch of water in a small saucepan. Cover the pan and place over high heat.

Wash the broccoli flowerets and trim lengthwise into small equal-sized pieces. When the water boils, put the broccoli into the pan.

Cover and steam for 30 seconds. Drain and rinse under cold water. Pat dry.

Wash the celery and remove the tough strings. Cut into diagonal slices about $\frac{1}{4}$ inch thick. Set aside.

Put the oil in a wok or a heavy 10-inch skillet with sloping sides. Crush the garlic with a heavy knife and remove the skin. Cut the gingerroot into 6 pieces and place it in the wok with the garlic. Heat the wok until the oil is hot and the garlic and gingerroot are lightly browned. Remove them and discard. Add the broccoli and celery to the wok. Toss with Chinese stir-frying utensils or two large spoons, for 1 minute. Remove from heat. Add the bean sprouts and the sauce. Toss for 30 seconds or until the sauce coats the vegetables. Eat right away.

Cauliflower and Green Bean Stir-Fry

Preparation time: about 5 minutes
Portions: 2
Calories per portion: 55

SAUCE

$\frac{1}{4}$ teaspoon cornstarch
$\frac{1}{2}$ tablespoon dry sherry

$\frac{1}{2}$ tablespoon Homemade
   Chicken Stock (see Index)
$\frac{1}{2}$ teaspoon imported soy sauce

---

3 ounces cauliflower flowerets
3 ounces fresh green beans
1 ounce scallion, white and
   green part, trimmed of
   root end

1 small clove garlic
1 quarter-sized slice fresh
   gingerroot
1 teaspoon vegetable oil

Dissolve the cornstarch in the sherry. Add the chicken stock and soy sauce. Mix to combine.

Place a small, covered pan with 1 inch of water over high heat.

Wash the cauliflower pieces and trim lengthwise through the stem into small equal-sized pieces. When the water boils, put the cauliflower into the pan. Cover and steam for 30 seconds. Remove with a slotted spoon. Rinse under cold water, pat dry, and set aside.

Wash the beans and remove the ends. Slice the beans diagonally. Place the beans in the hot water and steam for 30 seconds. Remove with a slotted spoon. Rinse under cold water, pat dry, and set aside.

Cut the scallion into thin 1-inch-long julienne strips.

Crush the garlic clove with a heavy knife and remove the skin. Cut the gingerroot into 6 pieces. Heat the oil, garlic, and gingerroot in a wok or a heavy 10-inch skillet with sloping sides. Heat until very hot but not smoking. When the garlic and gingerroot are lightly browned, remove them and discard. Add the cauliflower and green beans to the wok. Toss with Chinese stir-frying utensils or two large spoons for 1 minute. Add the scallions and toss. Remove the wok from the heat. Add the sauce and toss for 30 seconds. Eat right away.

Zucchini e Pomodori Saltati (Stir-Sautéed Zucchini and Tomatoes)

This snack is an Italian version of stir frying—made with tender young zucchini and red ripe garden tomatoes.

Preparation time: about 10 minutes
Portions: 4
Calories per portion: 42

8 ounces young zucchini, about 1 inch in diameter	**2 teaspoons fresh basil leaves or oregano leaves**
8 ounces very ripe tomato	**1 clove garlic**
2 tablespoons grated imported Parmesan cheese, very loosely packed	**1 teaspoon virgin olive oil**
	¼ teaspoon kosher salt
	Freshly ground black pepper

Wash the zucchini and trim the stem end. Slice into ⅛-inch-wide circles. Halve the tomato. Squeeze gently to remove seeds. Discard the seeds and remove the core from the tomato top. Cut the tomato into small chunks.

Grate the Parmesan and set aside. If using basil leaves, roll them into a tight tube and slice thin. If using oregano, chop the leaves very fine. Set aside.

Crush the garlic with a heavy knife and remove the skin. Place the garlic with the olive oil in a wok or a heavy 10-inch skillet with sloping sides. Heat until the oil is hot and the garlic is light brown. Remove garlic and discard.

Put the sliced zucchini in the pan. With Chinese stir-frying utensils or two large spoons, toss the zucchini over high heat for 1 minute. Add the chopped tomatoes and toss for 1 minute more. Remove from heat and toss with basil or oregano. Season with salt and pepper. Put on plates and garnish with the Parmesan cheese. This snack can be eaten hot or at room temperature. If it is refrigerated, bring to room temperature before eating.

HOT VEGETABLE SNACKS

Celery Steamed in Chicken Stock and Caraway

Preparation time: about 7 minutes
Portions: 1
Calories per portion: 31

¼ cup Homemade Chicken
   Stock (see Index)
4 ounces celery, trimmed of
   root end and leaves

¹⁄₁₆ teaspoon caraway seeds
Pinch of kosher salt

Place the chicken stock in a small saucepan over medium heat. Scrub the celery and cut into ¼-inch diagonal half-moons. Crush the caraway seeds in a mortar and pestle until they are medium-fine. Put the celery and the caraway into the chicken stock. Cover the pan and cook over medium high heat. When the stock boils, toss the celery frequently by lifting the pan from the stove and shaking it to redistribute the celery. Cook until the celery is bright green and still very crisp (about 4–5 minutes). Season with a pinch of salt, if desired. Eat right away or cool, refrigerate, and then gently reheat.

Dilly Carrot Puree

Preparation time: about 25 minutes
Portions: 1
Calories per portion: 73

6 ounces carrot, trimmed of stem ends

½ teaspoon fresh dill leaves
Pinch of kosher salt

Place 1 inch of water in a small deep saucepan. Cover and place over high heat.

Scrub the carrot well. Cut into 3-inch lengths. When the water boils, place an adjustable, nonaluminum steamer rack into the pan and place the carrots on the rack. Cover and reduce the heat to medium high. Steam the carrots until a sharp knife can easily be inserted into the carrots (about 20 minutes).

Chop the dill and set aside.

Remove the carrots and puree in a blender, food processor fitted with the steel blade, or through a food mill. Season with a pinch of kosher salt and garnish with the chopped dill. If making this snack in advance, cool the puree, then refrigerate. Reheat gently, stirring constantly, in a small saucepan. Garnish with the dill and eat.

Zucchini Toss

This delicate zucchini snack also makes a fine vegetable accompaniment for a fish dinner.

Preparation time: about 5 minutes
Portions: 1
Calories per portion: 21

4 ounces zucchini, firm and glossy
¼ ounce scallion, white part only, trimmed of root end

Freshly ground black pepper
1 lemon wedge

Scrub the zucchini and trim the stem end. Shred on the coarse side of a vegetable grater. Cut the scallion piece into julienne strips. Mix with the zucchini.

Place the vegetables in a small cold skillet and toss over high heat for 2–3 minutes until the zucchini is bright green and hot. Garnish with 1–2 grinds of black pepper and the juice from the lemon wedge. Eat hot or at room temperature. If refrigerated, allow to come to room temperature before eating.

Sesame Asparagus

Preparation time: about 9 minutes
Portions: 6
Calories per portion: 13

1 pound asparagus
½ teaspoon sesame seeds
2 lime wedges

Fill a wide-bottomed sauté pan or Dutch skillet with 1 inch of water. Cover and place over high heat.

Wash the asparagus in cold water. Cut off and discard the woody portion at the base of the stalks. With a vegetable peeler or sharp knife, peel the stalks to just below the tips. Tie the asparagus in a bundle with kitchen twine.

When the water boils, place the asparagus in the pan. Cover and return the water to a boil, then reduce the heat to a simmer. Steam the asparagus until the stalks are tender but still firm when pierced with a sharp knife (about 8 minutes). Remove the asparagus with tongs. Cut the string and spread the asparagus on a towel to cool and drain.

Place the sesame seeds in a small cold skillet. Toast over medium-high heat, tossing occasionally, until golden brown. Place the asparagus on a platter. Sprinkle with the sesame seeds and lime juice. Eat immediately at room temperature or refrigerate. If refrigerated, allow asparagus to come to room temperature before eating.

Parmesan Brussels Sprouts

Preparation time: about 15 minutes
Portions: 4
Calories per portion: 49

13 ounces Brussels sprouts
2 tablespoons grated imported
   Parmesan cheese, very
   loosely packed
Freshly ground black pepper

Select a saucepan at least 4 inches deep and 10 inches wide. Fill it with 1–2 inches of water. Cover and set over high heat.

Wash the Brussels sprouts and remove and discard any discolored outer leaves. Trim the stem end of each sprout and cut a shallow cross into each end. When the water boils, place an adjustable nonaluminum steamer rack into the pan and place the Brussels sprouts on the rack. Reduce the heat so that the water is just simmering and steam the sprouts until tender but still firm when pierced with a sharp knife (about 13 minutes).

When the sprouts are cooked, transfer them to a bowl, saving the steaming water for soup. Sprinkle the sprouts with the grated Parmesan and 4–5 grinds of black pepper. Toss to coat all of the sprouts. These can be eaten hot, or cooled and refrigerated. If refrigerated, let them come to room temperature before eating.

Rosy Brussels Sprouts

Preparation time: about 20 minutes
Portions: 4
Calories per portion: 48

13 ounces Brussels sprouts   **¾ cup tomato juice**
1 medium clove garlic   **Freshly ground black pepper**

Fill a 4-inch-high, 10-inch-wide saucepan with about 2 inches of water. Cover and place over high heat.

Follow the procedure in the preceding recipe (Parmesan Brussels Sprouts) for cleaning and preparing the sprouts. Steam the sprouts for 10 minutes.

Chop the garlic very fine and place in a saucepan with the tomato juice. Simmer, covered, for 10 minutes.

Remove the Brussels sprouts and place in the pan with the tomato juice. Simmer, tossing frequently for about 10 minutes, until the tomato juice is reduced and has begun to coat the sprouts. Garnish with 4-5 grinds of black pepper. Eat hot or cool and refrigerate. Reheat the sprouts gently over low heat.

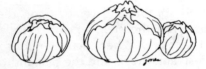

Provençal Vegetable Gratin

A luscious cheese custard sauce provides the crowning touch for this Provençal vegetable gratin. With a salad and crusty French bread, this dish becomes a delectable summertime meal.

Preparation time: about 10 minutes (with peppers already roasted)
Baking time: about 40 minutes
Portions: 8
Calories per portion: 77

1 teaspoon virgin olive oil
1 pound red peppers, roasted, cleaned, and cut into strips (see technique used in Roasted Red Pepper with Balsamic Vinegar; can be done several days in advance and refrigerated)

7 ounces yellow onion
1 pound ripe tomatoes
1½ tablespoons fresh or frozen oregano or ¾ teaspoon dried
Kosher salt
Freshly ground black pepper

CHEESE SAUCE

**4 ounces part-skim ricotta
 cheese
1 large egg
⅓ cup skim milk**

**3 tablespoons grated imported
 Parmesan cheese, very
 loosely packed
3–4 dashes of freshly ground
 white pepper**

Preheat the oven to 425° F. Grease a 10-inch oval gratin dish with the olive oil. Arrange the roasted pepper strips across the bottom of the dish and set aside.

Peel the onion and slice thin. Place in a heavy skillet with ¼ inch of water. Cover and set over high heat. When the water boils, remove the lid and toss the onions. Reduce the heat to medium and toss the onions until soft (about 10 minutes). If they start to brown, add a little water to the skillet.

Set a small pan of water, covered, over high heat. When it boils, remove from the heat and drop the tomatoes into the water for 45 seconds. Remove the tomatoes and rinse under cold water. Remove the core and skin with a sharp knife. Halve the tomatoes and gently squeeze out the seeds. Discard the seeds, core, and skins. Chop the tomatoes very fine with a heavy knife or in the food processor fitted with the steel blade. If using fresh oregano, chop it fine and mix with the tomatoes. If using dried oregano, crush it in a mortar and pestle and mix with the tomatoes.

To make the sauce and assemble the gratin: If the ricotta is wet, place it in the center of a clean cotton or linen towel. Wring it into a tight ball over a bowl or the sink. Blot with the dry corners of the towel until the excess moisture is removed and the ricotta holds together in a ball. Cream the ricotta in a small mixing bowl. Beat the egg in a small dish and add to the ricotta. Mix well to combine. Gradually add the skim milk and mix until smooth. Blend the grated Parmesan into the cheese sauce. Season with 3–4 dashes of freshly ground white pepper.

Sprinkle the pepper strips with salt and freshly ground pepper. Spread the onions over the peppers and season with salt and pepper. Spread the chopped tomatoes over the onions and sprinkle with salt and pepper. Pour the cheese sauce over the vegetables and spread evenly. (At this point the gratin can be refrigerated for up to

24 hours before baking. If baking from the refrigerator, the baking time will be slightly increased.)

Bake for 10 minutes, then reduce the heat to 375° F. Bake for 25–30 minutes more, until the top is puffy and brown. Remove from the oven and let the gratin sit for 5 minutes before serving. The gratin is good hot or at room temperature.

Hearts of Fennel Braised in Tomato Puree

Fennel is widely used in French and Italian cuisine but is relatively unknown to American cooks. Its mild anise flavor and crunchy celerylike texture make it a welcome addition to the vegetable repertoire. The fennel head looks like a short, fat bunch of celery topped with dark green lacy leaves.

Preparation time: about 30 minutes
Portions: 2
Calories per portion: 81

1 small clove garlic
12 ounces very ripe Italian
    plum tomatoes or 10
    ounces canned Italian
    plum tomatoes

¼ teaspoon kosher salt
3 grinds of fresh black pepper
20-ounce head of fennel

GARNISH

1 teaspoon fresh fennel leaves

Crush the garlic clove with a heavy knife. Lift off the skin and discard. Chop the garlic fine and set aside.

If using fresh tomatoes, remove the skin and seeds. If using canned tomatoes, remove the seeds and juice and save the juice for another recipe. (For both techniques, see recipe for Ratatouille.) Puree the tomatoes with the steel blade in a food processor blender or through a food mill. Combine with the chopped garlic in a small sauté pan or skillet that will be large enough to hold the fennel in a single layer. Season with salt and pepper.

Wash the fennel. Trim the bottom of the stalk and discard. Trim the thin stalks from the top. Set aside. Cut the head in half lengthwise. Place the fennel hearts in the tomato puree. Cover and place over medium heat. As soon as the puree starts to bubble, reduce the heat to a low simmer and cook, covered, for 20–25 minutes, until the fennel is tender when pierced with a sharp knife.

Trim the leaves from the fennel stalks that were set aside. Discard the stalks or dry them in a cool spot to use later for grilling fish. Wash and dry the leaves. Chop 1 teaspoon for garnishing the fennel hearts. Store the remaining leaves in a paper towel–lined plastic bag with some air holes punched into it.

Zucchini Crust Pizza

This unconventional pizza substitutes shredded zucchini for bread dough as a crust. The results are unconventionally delicious.

Preparation time: about 10 minutes
Baking time: about 30 minutes
Portions: 8 wedges
Calories per portion: 66

ZUCCHINI CRUST

1 pound 10 ounces small firm zucchini
½ ounce scallion, white and green part, trimmed of root end

½ ounce dry bread crumbs (see technique for making bread crumbs in Artichoke Stuffed with Ham and Cheese)
1 large egg

TOPPING

1¾ teaspoons fresh or frozen oregano leaves or ¾ teaspoon dried leaves

½ cup tomato puree
3 ounces part-skim mozzarella cheese

Preheat the oven to 350° F.

Scrub the zucchini in cold water, then pat dry. Cut off the stem ends and discard. Shred the zucchini on the coarse side of a vegetable grater. Set aside. Cut the scallion into ¾-inch-long pieces and then into julienne strips. Combine with the shredded zucchini and place in a cold 10-inch sauté pan. Place over high heat and toss the zucchini for about 5 minutes, until much of the moisture is cooked off. Drain the zucchini and set aside to cool slightly.

Squeeze as much moisture as possible from the zucchini. In a bowl, mix the zucchini with the bread crumbs. Beat the egg in a small bowl and add to the zucchini mixture. Toss to combine. Press the zucchini into an 11½-inch round pizza pan. With the hands or the back of a large spoon, press the mixture evenly to cover the bottom of the pan. Press the mixture up slightly around the edges to form a raised edge. Place in the oven and bake for 5 minutes.

If using fresh oregano, chop the leaves very fine. If using dried oregano, crush the leaves in a mortar and pestle or between the fingers. Mix the oregano with the tomato puree. Set aside. Shred the cheese on the coarse side of a vegetable grater and set aside.

Remove the crust from the oven and spread the tomato puree and oregano evenly over the top of the crust. Sprinkle the cheese evenly over the top and return the pizza to the oven.

Bake for 25 minutes or until the top is brown and the cheese is bubbly. Remove from the oven and allow to sit for 5 minutes. Run a small sharp knife between the side crust and the pan, then cut into 8 wedges. Eat right away.

Cauliflower in Mustard Sauce

Preparation time: about 8 minutes
Portions: 2
Calories per portion: 44

6 ounces cauliflower flowerets

SAUCE

2 ounces low-fat cottage cheese

1 teaspoon Dijon or horseradish mustard

GARNISH

**½ teaspoon summer savory or
   Italian parsley**

Fill a saucepan that is at least 4–5 inches deep and 8 inches in diameter with 1–2 inches of water. Cover and set the pan over high heat.

Wash the cauliflower. Trim the flowerets into pieces of equal size. When the water boils, set a nonaluminum adjustable steamer rack into the pan. Reduce the heat so the water is cooking at a brisk simmer. Lay the cauliflower pieces on the steamer rack in a single layer. Cover with the lid and steam until the cauliflower is tender but still firm (about 7 minutes).

While the cauliflower is steaming, cream the cottage cheese by hand in a blender or in the bowl of a food processor fitted with the steel blade. Process until smooth. Add the mustard and mix. Place the sauce in a small bowl. Chop the savory or parsley leaves and set aside.

When the cauliflower is cooked, remove and place in the bowl with the sauce. Toss gently to coat the cauliflower with the sauce. Garnish with the chopped herb. This snack can be eaten hot or cold. If refrigerated, allow to come to room temperature before eating.

Mushrooms Stewed with Rosemary

This dish is a delicious accompaniment to chicken or fish.

Preparation time: about 8 minutes
Portions: 3
Calories per portion: 32

**8 ounces firm white
   mushrooms**
**½ teaspoon fresh or frozen
   rosemary leaves or ⅛
   teaspoon dried**

1 teaspoon virgin olive oil
Pinch of kosher salt
2 grinds of black pepper

Clean the mushrooms with a mushroom brush or damp cloth. Trim the ends and discard. Slice the mushrooms. Chop the rosemary very fine. Warm the olive oil in an 8-inch skillet. Coat the bottom of the skillet with the oil. Place the sliced mushrooms and chopped rosemary in the skillet. Cover with a heavy lid. Cook over medium heat for 1–2 minutes, until the mushrooms start to exude moisture. Remove the lid and turn the heat up to high. Toss over high heat until liquid is evaporated (about 3 minutes). Season with salt and pepper. Eat right away or cool the mushrooms and refrigerate. To reheat, place the mushrooms in a small saucepan and toss gently over low heat.

Wilted Romaine with Toasted Sesame Seeds

An important part of keeping a diet interesting is preparing foods in unexpected ways. Most people enjoy crisp romaine in a salad, but it can also be an appetizing cooked vegetable.

Preparation time: 5 minutes
Portions: 1
Calories per portion: 35

6 ounces romaine (if using
   large outer leaves, weigh
   them after trimming and
   discarding the pulpy
   spines)
¼ teaspoon sesame seeds

Wash the romaine leaves in cold water. Tear the leaves into bite-sized pieces. With the water clinging to the leaves, lift them from the water into a small nonaluminum saucepan (don't add any water). Cover and place over medium-high heat. When the water on the bottom leaves becomes hot (about 1 minute) remove the lid and toss the leaves. Replace the lid and steam for about 1 more minute, until leaves are wilted but still bright green.

While the leaves are steaming, place the sesame seeds in a small heavy skillet over medium-high heat. Toast the seeds, tossing occasionally, until they are golden brown. Remove from the heat.

When the leaves are steamed, drain and toss to remove excess moisture. Sprinkle with the toasted sesame seeds and eat right away.

Ratatouille (French Vegetable Stew)

This versatile French vegetable stew tastes great at any temperature. As well as being a delicious side dish, Ratatouille can be used to fill crepes or omelets. Topped with some grated cheese and run under a broiler, it makes a lovely main course.

Preparation time: about 30 minutes
Cooking time: about 1 hour
Portions: 20
Calories per portion: 76

1 pound eggplant
1 teaspoon kosher salt
10 ounces small firm zucchini
10 ounces green peppers
10 ounces yellow onions
14 ounces very ripe plum tomatoes or 1 28-ounce can tomatoes, drained
2 cloves garlic
2 tablespoons fresh thyme or 2 teaspoons dried

2 tablespoons fresh parsley stems
2 tablespoons fresh tarragon leaves or 2 teaspoons dried
1 bay leaf
3 tablespoons virgin olive oil
1 teaspoon kosher salt
½ teaspoon freshly ground black pepper

Wash all the vegetables. Cut the stem end from the eggplant and cut into ½-inch-thick lengthwise slices. Stack the slices together and slice into ½-inch-wide strips. Cut through the stacked strips at ½-inch intervals to make ½-inch cubes. Place the eggplant cubes in a nonaluminum colander and sprinkle with 1 teaspoon kosher salt. Toss to coat all the cubes with salt. Place the colander over a bowl and set aside.

Place a covered 2-quart saucepan of water over high heat.

Cut the stem ends from the zucchini. Cut in half lengthwise and then into ½-inch chunks. Place the zucchini in a 4- to 6-quart heavy nonaluminum Dutch oven or saucepan. Set aside.

Cut the tops from the green peppers. Cut in half and remove the seeds and ribs. Cut into ½-inch squares and place with the zucchini.

Peel the onions and slice in half through the stem. Lay each cut half on its flat side and make cuts with a sharp knife at ½-inch intervals that run downward from the stem ends. Now make cuts at ½-inch intervals that are perpendicular to the first cuts. Slice down through the onion to the flat side at ½-inch intervals. Place the chopped onion with the zucchini and peppers.

When the water boils, turn off the heat and place the tomatoes in the water for 45 seconds. Remove and rinse with cold water. Using a sharp knife, remove the cores and the skin. Halve the tomatoes and squeeze gently to release seeds. Discard cores, seeds, and skin. Chop the tomato flesh coarsely and add to the pan with the other vegetables. (If using canned tomatoes, remove the tomatoes from the can one at a time, slitting the side of the tomato open as you do so. With a knife or a finger, scrape the seeds into the can. When all the tomatoes have been lifted out and seeded, chop them coarsely and place in the pan with the vegetables. Strain the seeds from the juice and refrigerate the juice for drinking or use in another recipe.)

Smash the garlic cloves with a heavy knife. Lift off the skin and discard. Chop the garlic fine and add to the pan. Prepare a *bouquet garni* with the thyme, parsley, tarragon, and bay leaf (see technique in Chapter 1). If using fresh tarragon, reserve 1 tablespoon to garnish the finished Ratatouille.

Rinse the eggplant cubes under cold running water, then pat dry with a towel. Add to the pan. Drizzle the olive oil over the vegetables and toss. Place the *bouquet garni* in the center of the vegetables. Cover the pan and place over medium heat. Bring the vegetables to a rapid simmer, then lower the heat to a slow simmer. Simmer for about 1 hour, stirring occasionally, until the vegetables are very tender. Remove from the heat and take out the *bouquet garni,* pressing it against the inside of the pan with a large spoon to extract the juice. Discard the *bouquet garni.* Season with salt and pepper. Serve immediately or cool and refrigerate for up to a week. If using fresh tarragon, chop it for garnish and sprinkle on top of the Ratatouille before eating.

Eggplant Pizza Rounds

Preparation time: about 45 minutes
Portions: 6
Calories per portion: 63

1 12-ounce or 2 6-ounce
   eggplants of uniform width
1 teaspoon kosher salt
1½ teaspoons fresh oregano or
   ¾ teaspoon dried
½ cup tomato puree

¼ teaspoon kosher salt
2 grinds of black pepper
3 ounces part-skim mozzarella
   cheese
1 teaspoon virgin olive oil

Wash and dry the eggplant. Trim the stem end and discard. Cut into ¾-inch-thick slices. Sprinkle both sides of the slices with kosher salt and lay on paper towels to drain for 30 minutes.

If using fresh oregano, chop the leaves very fine. If using dried, crush the leaves in a mortar and pestle or between fingers.

Mix the oregano with the tomato puree, salt, and pepper. Shred the mozzarella on the coarse side of a vegetable grater. Set aside.

After the eggplant slices have drained for 30 minutes, rinse them quickly under cold running water, then pat dry. Very lightly brush the broiler pan with olive oil. Position the pan about 5 inches from the heat source. Lay the slices on the broiler pan and broil until light brown (about 5–6 minutes). Turn and brown the other side (about 5–6 minutes). Spoon the sauce on top of the eggplant slices and cover with the cheese. Broil for about 5 minutes or until the cheese is brown and bubbly. Remove from the broiler and eat right away.

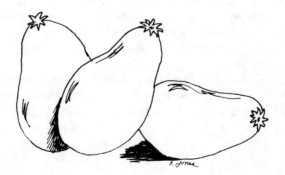

Spaghetti Squash Parmesan

Spaghetti squash not only tastes great; it's also fun to cook. The golden flesh unfurls into long strands resembling spaghetti.

Preparation time: about 15 minutes
Baking time: about 1 hour
Portions: 8
Calories per portion: 81

1 spaghetti squash,
    approximately 3¾ pounds
2 tablespoons grated imported
    Parmesan cheese, very
    loosely packed
Freshly ground black pepper

Preheat the oven to 350° F.

Wash and dry the squash. Place it in a shallow baking pan and put into the oven. Bake the squash for 1 hour or until a sharp knife inserted in the stem end comes out easily. During the baking, rotate the squash several times so it bakes evenly. Remove the squash from the oven and let it sit for 10 minutes.

Cut the squash in half lengthwise with a sharp knife. Scoop out the pulpy center and the seeds. Set aside. Discard the pulp and seeds or save the seeds to use in a recipe such as Roasted Squash or Pumpkin Seeds (see Index).

With a fork or large spoon, scrape ¼-inch layers from the hollow where the seeds were. The squash will come away in strands resembling spaghetti. Continue until you reach the rind, then repeat with the other half. At this point the squash can be cooled and refrigerated for several days.

To serve: Grate the Parmesan cheese and set aside. Toss the squash over low heat in a saucepan for 2–3 minutes. When it is hot, sprinkle with the grated cheese and 2–3 grinds of black pepper. Eat right away.

Broccoli Blossoms with Broccoli Puree

This broccoli snack doubles as a tasty side dish with roast lamb or beef.

Preparation time: about 10 minutes
Portions: 2
Calories per portion: 78

14 ounces broccoli   **1 teaspoon lemon juice**
1 ounce yellow onion   **Dash of white pepper**
1 teaspoon unsalted butter   **Pinch of kosher salt**

Place an inch of water in a 3-quart saucepan. Cover the pan and place over high heat. Wash the broccoli. Trim the base and peel the stem. Cut the flowerets from the broccoli stem with about 1 inch of the stem left attached to the flowerets. Cut the flowerets into portions of equal size, keeping the flower shape intact. Set aside. Chop the stem into small chunks. If there are more flowers than stems, put some of the flowers into the stem pile to make equal portions. Chop the onion into fine pieces and place with the broccoli stems.

When the water boils, place the stem pile with the onion into the pan. Cover and return to the boil. Reduce heat and steam until tender (about 5 minutes). Remove with a slotted spoon and lay on paper towels. Add more water to the pan, if necessary, to bring the level back to 1 inch. Set over medium heat.

Place the cooked stems and onions in a blender or the bowl of a food processor fitted with a steel blade. Puree, scraping down the sides of the bowl as necessary, until the mixture is smooth. Or puree through the fine disc of a food mill.

Bring the water back to a boil. Place the flowerets in the pan. Cover and cook for 1 minute. Drain the cooking liquid into a bowl and save it for later use in soup. Lay the flowerets on paper towels to drain.

Mix the butter, lemon juice, pepper, and salt with the puree. Place on two small dishes. Surround with the broccoli flowers for dipping. Serve right away.

Beet Greens with Lemon

These greens make a delightful side dish with roast or grilled pork or chicken.

Preparation time: about 8 minutes
Portions: 4
Calories per portion: 29

1 pound beet greens (the amount of greens on 2 pounds of fresh beets; see Pickled Beets)

Kosher salt
Freshly ground black pepper
4 lemon wedges

Wash the greens in cold water and remove the hard red spines.

Lift the greens from the water. Do not shake dry but place them in a heavy nonaluminum pan in which the greens fit tightly. Cover and cook over medium-high heat. After 1 minute, lift the lid and toss the greens. Cover and cook for 2–3 minutes more, until the greens are bright green and just wilted. Drain and toss to remove excess moisture. (Save the liquid for soup.)

Sprinkle each portion lightly with salt and freshly ground black pepper. Garnish with a wedge of lemon to squeeze over the greens. These greens can be eaten hot or cold. If they are refrigerated, bring them to room temperature before eating.

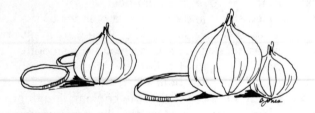

STUFFED VEGETABLE SNACKS

Most of these recipes are so versatile that they can be enjoyed at any temperature. With the addition of a tossed salad and bread, many of them make a satisfying light meal.

Stuffed Peppers with Brown Rice

Preparation time: about 10 minutes
Baking time: about 35 minutes
Portions: 4
Calories per portion: 105

4 4-ounce green bell peppers
2 ounces yellow onion
1 small clove garlic
4 ounces ripe tomato
**2 teaspoons fresh oregano or ½
teaspoon dried**
**2 ounces part-skim mozzarella
cheese**

6 ounces cooked brown rice
Dash of cayenne pepper
**⅛ teaspoon freshly ground
black pepper**
½ teaspoon kosher salt

Preheat the oven to 375° F. Place a 2-quart pan of water, covered, over high heat.

Wash the peppers and slice the tops. Reserve. With a sharp knife or spoon, scoop out the seeds and the white ribs from the peppers. Discard. Blanch the peppers in the boiling water for 3 minutes, then remove. Turn upside down on a towel to drain.

Chop the onion and garlic very fine and place in a small nonstick skillet. Cook gently over low heat for 5 minutes, stirring often. If onion sticks to the pan or starts to brown, add a few drops of water.

Cut the tomato in half and squeeze gently over a bowl to remove the seeds. Discard the seeds. Remove the tomato core and discard. Chop the tomato into small pieces.

If using fresh oregano, chop it very fine. If using dried oregano, crush the leaves in a mortar and pestle or between fingers.

Grate the cheese on the coarse side of a vegetable grater.

In a small bowl combine the rice, onion, garlic, tomato, and seasonings. Mix in the cheese. Scoop the stuffing into the pepper shells and cover with the reserved pepper tops. Choose an oven-proof dish in which the peppers will fit tightly. Place the peppers in the dish with ¼ inch of hot water.

Place the dish in the oven and bake for about 35 minutes. Uncover the peppers for the last 5 minutes of baking to brown the tops. Remove from the oven and allow to sit for 5 minutes before eating. Or cool the peppers and refrigerate. Allow to come to room temperature before eating.

Zucchini Ripieni (Italian Stuffed Zucchini)

This recipe is an adaptation of an old Italian favorite of mine. By substituting lean pork and my own herb mixture for the Italian sausage, and by cutting the amount of cheese and eliminating olive oil, I was able to reduce the calorie count to less than one-quarter of the original. And the new version tastes just as good. It proves that with a little ingenuity our favorite high-calorie recipes can be calorie-trimmed with no sacrifice of taste.

Preparation time: about 15 minutes
Baking time: 45 minutes
Portions: 16
Calories per portion: 56

8 ounces small firm zucchini (about 2 zucchini)
3 ounces lean pork loin, trimmed of all visible fat
4 ounces tomato
¼ ounce yellow onion
1 small clove garlic

1 ounce part-skim mozzarella cheese
1 tablespoon grated imported Parmesan cheese, very loosely packed
¼ teaspoon fennel seeds
¼ teaspoon kosher salt
4 grinds of black pepper

Preheat the oven to 400° F.

Scrub the zucchini and cut the stem ends off. Cut in half lengthwise. With a melon baller or spoon, scoop out the center, leaving a ¼-inch shell. Chop the scooped-out flesh and place in a bowl. Set the shells aside.

Cut the pork into small cubes and place in a meat grinder or food processor fitted with a steel blade. Process until finely ground. Or chop the pork into small pieces with a heavy chef's knife. Add to the bowl with the zucchini.

Cut the tomato in half and squeeze out the seeds. Remove the core. Discard the core and the seeds. Chop the tomato flesh into fine pieces and add to the bowl.

Chop the onion and garlic very fine and add to the bowl. Grate the mozzarella and Parmesan and add to the bowl. Coarsely crush the fennel seeds in a mortar and pestle. Add the salt and pepper and mix the seasonings to combine. With a spoon or a hand combine the ingredients in the mixing bowl. Sprinkle the spices over the mixture and mix to incorporate them evenly with the stuffing.

Select an ovenproof baking dish in which the zucchini will fit tightly. Place ¼ inch of hot water in the pan. Place the zucchini in the pan and fill the hollows with the stuffing mixture. Place in the oven and bake for 45 minutes. If the tops start to brown too quickly, cover loosely with aluminum foil. Remove from the oven and cut into 16 equal pieces. This snack is delicious eaten hot or at room temperature. If refrigerated, allow to come to room temperature before eating.

To make Zucchini Ripieni as a party hors d'oeuvre: Cut the zucchini into 16 discs. With a melon baller scoop part of the center of each disc out and chop. Follow the directions for making the stuffing. Fill each disc with an equal amount of stuffing. Bake for about 35 minutes, until nicely browned. These can be assembled in advance, refrigerated for up to 24 hours, then baked right before serving.

Artichoke Stuffed with Ham and Cheese

This artichoke can be stuffed in advance, covered tightly, and refrigerated for up to 24 hours before baking. It makes a stunning main course for a luncheon or brunch.

Preparation time: about 10 minutes
Baking time: 45 minutes
Portions: 2
Calories per portion: 124

½ **lemon**
1 12-ounce artichoke

STUFFING

½ **ounce completely lean ham**   **1 ounce low-fat cottage cheese**
¼ **ounce dry bread crumbs**   **3 grinds of black pepper**
1 tablespoon grated imported
    Parmesan cheese, very
    loosely packed

Preheat the oven to 375° F.

Fill a 3-cup bowl with cold water and squeeze the lemon juice into the water. Drop the lemon into the water and set aside. Wash the artichoke and cut off the stem. With a heavy knife cut off the top inch of the artichoke. With the fingers peel off the first several layers of leaves at the base of the artichoke. When the leaves start to show a color gradation of dark green at the top and lighter green at the bottom, use kitchen shears to cut off just the top part of each leaf. Continue toward the top until all the leaves are trimmed.

With the fingers of one hand, spread the center leaves gently apart to reveal the cream-colored and purple prickly inner leaves. Remove these by pulling them out with the fingers of the other hand. With a sharp spoon, scrape the fuzzy choke away from the heart of the artichoke and discard. Rinse under cold water. Rub the artichoke all over with the lemon half and then place the lemon in the center of the artichoke. Place the artichoke in the lemon water and set aside.

To prepare the stuffing: Chop the ham into fine pieces. Place in a small mixing bowl and combine with the bread crumbs, Parmesan cheese, and cottage cheese. (To made bread crumbs from the French Bread recipe in this book, cut any stale bread into chunks and let sit on a plate, covered only by a towel, for two days. When the bread is very hard, grind in a food processor fitted with a steel blade or in a blender. The bread crumbs may be stored for several months in an airtight tin in a cool spot.) Season with pepper to taste. Select a small high-sided baking dish (one that will hold the artichoke upright as it bakes). Cover the bottom of the dish with 1/4 inch of hot water.

Remove the artichoke from the water and remove the lemon from the center. Pat the artichoke dry. With the fingers of one hand, hold the center leaves open. Spoon the stuffing into the center cavity. When it is full, spread open the leaves nearest to the center and place stuffing between them. Continue until all the stuffing is used.

Place the artichoke in the baking dish and cover with aluminum foil. Bake for 40 minutes. Remove the foil and bake until the artichoke is lightly browned on top. Remove from the oven and let the artichoke sit for 10 minutes. Cut in half lengthwise. The artichoke can be eaten hot or cold. If refrigerated, allow the artichoke to come to room temperature before eating.

Baked Tomato Stuffed with Cheese and Spinach

Preparation time: about 5 minutes
Baking time: about 20 minutes
Portions: 1
Calories per portion: 87

1 4-ounce tomato, ripe but firm
3 ounces spinach leaves,
   trimmed of stems and
   spines
1 ounce low-fat cottage cheese

1 tablespoon grated imported
   Romano cheese, very
   loosely packed
2–3 grinds of black pepper

Preheat the oven to 350° F.

Wash the tomato and cut off the top. Set aside. With a finger, scoop out the seeds and discard. With a spoon, scoop out the flesh, leaving a ¼-inch wall. Chop the flesh very fine and place in a small bowl.

Wash the spinach leaves and place them in a small nonaluminum pan with the water clinging to the leaves (don't add any water). Cover and cook for 1–2 minutes, tossing once, until the spinach is wilted. Drain and squeeze as dry as possible. Chop very fine and add to the tomato bowl.

Mix the remaining ingredients with the tomato and spinach. Fill the tomato with the stuffing and place in a small narrow baking dish with about ¼ inch of hot water in the bottom of the dish. Place the tomato top over the stuffing and put the dish in the oven.

Bake for about 20 minutes, until the tomato is soft. During the last 5 minutes of baking, remove the tomato top so the stuffing can brown. This snack can be eaten hot or at room temperature. If refrigerated, bring back to room temperature before eating.

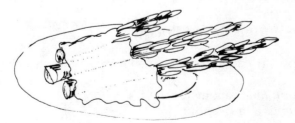

Savory Stuffed Onion

Preparation time: about 6 minutes
Baking time: about 1 hour
Portions: 1
Calories per portion: 136

1 6-ounce yellow onion
½ teaspoon unsalted butter
1 tablespoon Italian parsley
  leaves

2 fresh or frozen sage leaves
½ ounce Gruyère cheese
Pinch of kosher salt
3 grinds of black pepper

Preheat the oven to 375° F.

Peel the onion and slice off the root end so it sits flat. Slice off the top of the onion and, with a spoon or melon baller, scoop out the onion flesh. Leave ¼-inch-thick onion walls.

Chop the onion flesh very fine. Melt the butter in a small skillet and add the chopped onion. Stew the onion over low heat until soft, about 5 minutes.

Chop the herbs and grate the cheese. Combine with the onions and salt and pepper. Stuff tightly into the hollow onion. Place in a small ovenproof dish that is half full of hot water. Cover loosely with foil and place in the oven.

After 30 minutes, remove the foil and bake for another 30 minutes. If the onion starts to brown too quickly, reduce the heat to 350° F. Remove from the oven and let sit for 10 minutes before eating. Spoon some of the cooking juice over the onion; the rest can be saved for soup.

Cheddar-Stuffed Baked Potato

Eat the potato skin and get all the vitamins from this tasty snack.

Preparation time: about 10 minutes
Baking time: about 1 hour
Portions: 2
Calories per portion: 97

1 6-ounce baking potato
½ ounce cheddar cheese
¼ teaspoon fresh or frozen
    chives, basil, or tarragon

1 tablespoon skim milk
Dash of kosher salt

Preheat the oven to 375° F.

Scrub the potato and pat dry. Pierce the potato several times on all sides with the tines of a fork. Place the potato on a baking rack in the center of the oven and bake for 45–50 minutes, until the flesh feels soft when squeezed.

While the potato is roasting, shred the cheese on a vegetable grater or chop fine with a knife. Chop the herb and set aside.

When the potato is cooked, remove from the oven and lower the oven temperature to 350° F. With a sharp knife, slice the top lengthwise from the potato. Scrape the flesh from the top and bottom. Mash the flesh with a potato masher or potato ricer. With an electric mixer or whisk, beat in the milk until very smooth. Season with salt and mix in the cheese and herb. Spoon the potato puree back into the shell and place on a small baking dish. Return to the oven for 10 minutes to heat the stuffing. If a browner top is desired, run under the broiler for 2–3 minutes. Remove from the oven and cut into two portions.

Herb-Stuffed Mushrooms

These mushrooms make a great party hors d'oeuvre. Prepare them in advance and bake just before serving.

Preparation time: about 5 minutes
Baking time: about 20 minutes
Portions: 4
Calories per portion: 28

4 large mushrooms (about 8
    ounces)
1 teaspoon Italian parsley
    leaves
1 small clove garlic
¼ ounce bread crumbs (see
    Artichoke Stuffed with
    Ham and Cheese)

Juice from 1 lemon wedge
1 teaspoon unsalted butter at
    room temperature
Freshly ground black pepper

Preheat the oven to 350° F.

Clean the mushrooms with a damp mushroom brush or damp cloth. Carefully remove the stems by pulling them out. (Save the stems for soup or a stuffing.)

Chop the parsley leaves and set aside. Crush the garlic clove with a mortar and pestle. Remove the skin and discard. Crush the clove, combining the remaining ingredients in the process. Season with 1–2 grinds of black pepper.

Divide the stuffing into 4 mushroom caps and press down. Wrap tightly in aluminum foil. (At this point, the mushroom caps can be refrigerated.)

Place 2 teaspoons of water into the foil with the mushrooms. Rewrap and bake in a preheated 350° F. oven for 18 minutes. Open the foil and place the mushrooms under the broiler until brown (2–3 minutes). Spoon the juice over the top before eating.

Whipped Sweet Potato in the Shell

Slow baking converts the starch in the sweet potato into sugar, so no added sugar is needed. This sweet potato recipe makes a much more elegant accompaniment to the Thanksgiving turkey than canned sweet potatoes buried under mounds of brown sugar and marshmallow whip.

Preparation time: about 4 minutes
Baking time: about 1 hour
Portions: 2
Calories per portion: 83

1 5-ounce sweet potato
½ tablespoon skim milk
Freshly grated nutmeg

Preheat the oven to 375° F.

Scrub the sweet potato and pat dry. Place the potato on a baking rack in the center of the oven and bake until the flesh feels soft when pressed (about 50 minutes).

Remove the potato from the oven and cut a long oval slice from one side. With a spoon, scoop out the flesh from the bottom and the top slice. Whip by hand or with an electric mixer, gradually adding the milk, until the puree is smooth. Grate nutmeg to taste into the puree and mix. Spoon the puree back into the shell and return to the oven for 10 minutes to heat through. For a fancier presentation, the puree can be piped through a decorative pastry tip into the shell.

3
Fabulous Fruit Snacks

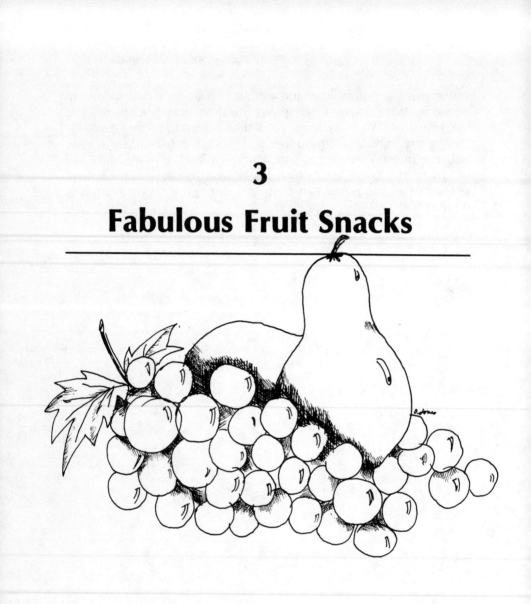

The best way for a dieter to enjoy fruit is straight from Mother Nature—in self-contained little packages of sweetness, flavor, vitamins, and natural fiber. (See Chapter 1 for information on selecting and ripening fruit.) Unadulterated fruit, of course, will have fewer calories than fruit with added condiments. But because variety is such an important aspect of a successful weight-loss diet, from time to time we will jazz things up a bit.

Fresh fruit compotes, with the addition of spices, herbs, wine, citrus juices, or yogurt provide an added flavor dimension to luscious fresh fruits without too high a toll in additional calories.

Tasty, refreshing fruit snacks can be incorporated into meal plans as appetizers, salads, and desserts. Like some of the vegetable snacks in the preceding chapter, many of these fruit compotes are at their flavor peak at room temperature or just slightly chilled.

UNCOOKED FRUIT SNACKS

Apple Cider Gel

Preparation time: about 10 minutes
Chilling time: at least 4 hours
Portions: 8
Calories per portion: 87

2 envelopes unflavored gelatin
½ cup cold water
4 cups pure apple juice or cider

12 ounces apples (2 6-ounce apples)

Sprinkle the gelatin over ½ cup cold water in a heatproof measuring cup. Place the cup in a pan of hot water to melt (about 4–5 minutes), double boiler style. The gelatin should look clear and no longer grainy.

In a mixing bowl combine the gelatin with 4 cups apple juice. Mix well. Cover and refrigerate until it starts to set to the consistency of egg white (about 2 hours). Check from time to time because some refrigerators may be colder than others.

Wash the apples and cut into quarters. Remove the cores and slice the apples. Pour about ¼ of the apple gel into a 6-cup mold or dish. Line with a layer of apple slices. Cover with several spoons of the apple gel. Continue making layers of gel and apples until all the apples are used and the top is covered with gel. (There should be about 4 layers, depending on the dimensions of the mold.) Cover and chill for several hours or overnight.

If desired, this gel can be unmolded. Oil the dish with 1 teaspoon of vegetable oil and prepare as above. To unmold, follow technique in Gazpacho Aspic.

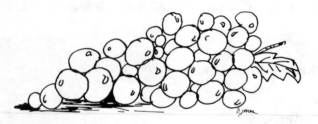

Arctic Grapes

This is a super dessert for a lazy, hot summer night.

Preparation time: about 1 minute
Freezing time: about 3 hours
Portions: 1
Calories per portion: 76

4 ounces seedless white grapes

Wash and dry the grapes. Place them in a plastic bag and put in the freezer for 3 hours or until frozen through.

To eat, let each grape melt on the tongue into a pool of light, exquisite grape sherbet.

For best texture, eat the grapes as soon as possible after they are frozen.

Minted Oranges

As a breakfast fruit, this snack can be a soothing beginning to your daily routine.

Preparation time: about 5 minutes
Marinating time: at least 2 hours
Portions: 1
Calories per portion: 79

1 7½-ounce orange
1 teaspoon fresh mint leaves

Peel the orange and cut into sections. Place in a glass or ceramic bowl. Chop the mint leaves and stir into the oranges. Cover the dish tightly and put in the refrigerator to marinate for at least 2 hours or as long as 24.

Rum-Spiked Pears

Preparation time: about 5 minutes
Marinating time: several hours
Portions: 2
Calories per portion: 83

10 ounces pears, very ripe (2 5-ounce pears)
1 teaspoon light or dark 80-proof rum

Freshly grated or ground cinnamon

Wash the pears and cut into quarters. Remove the cores. Slice the pears thin and immediately toss with the rum in a nonaluminum bowl. Dust with cinnamon, toss gently, and dust again. Cover with plastic wrap and marinate in the refrigerator for several hours before eating. Let the pears sit at room temperature 10–15 minutes before eating.

Cantaloupe Balls in Port Wine

Cantaloupe Balls in Port Wine serve as an excellent light first course for a dinner party.

Preparation time: about 5 minutes
Marinating time: several hours
Portions: 20
Calories per portion: 4

1 1-pound cantaloupe
1 tablespoon port or Madeira
   wine
Freshly grated nutmeg

Cut the cantaloupe in half. Scoop out and discard the seeds. With a large melon baller, scoop out 20 melon balls. (The melon balls should weigh 7 ounces.) In a glass dish, sprinkle with the port or Madeira wine and then dust all the balls lightly with freshly grated nutmeg.

Cover with plastic and refrigerate for several hours before serving. Let the melon sit at room temperature 15 minutes before eating.

Grape and Strawberry Salad

Preparation time: about 10 minutes
Marinating time: several hours
Portions: 8
Calories per portion: 66

1 pint very ripe but firm   **1 pound seedless white grapes**
   strawberries   **¼ cup dry white wine**

Wash and hull the strawberries. Cut into thin slices. Wash and halve the grapes. Place the fruit in a glass or ceramic dish and pour the wine over the top. Toss gently. Cover and marinate at room temperature for 2 hours. Twenty minutes before eating, refresh the fruit by chilling in the refrigerator.

Cranberry Raisin Relish

Cranberries and raisins combine in a wonderful relish to serve with roast chicken, turkey, or pork.

Preparation time: about 3 minutes
Marinating time: at least 24 hours
Portions: 6
Calories per portion: 68

12 ounces fresh cranberries
2 ounces dark raisins

¾ cup freshly squeezed orange juice (juice from about 2 medium oranges)

Wash the cranberries well under cold water. Pat dry.

In the bowl of a food processor fitted with a steel blade, place the cranberries and raisins. Chop into small pieces. The cranberries and raisins can also be chopped with a heavy chef's knife.

Place the chopped fruits in a bowl. Squeeze the orange juice and mix with the fruits. Cover and marinate in the refrigerator for 24 hours or longer. Toss several times while the fruit is marinating.

Papaya with Lemon or Lime

The luscious deep yellow flesh of the papaya makes a wonderful snack any time of the day. If the fruit's skin is green when purchased, allow it to ripen to a yellowish green before eating.

Preparation time: about 1 minute
Portions: 4
Calories per portion: 45

1 ripe papaya, approximately 1¼ pounds

4 lemon or lime wedges

Wash and dry the fruit. Cut into 4 lengthwise quarters. Remove the seeds with a spoon and discard. Garnish each wedge with the juice of a lemon or lime wedge.

If eating 1 portion of papaya and refrigerating the rest, wrap the pieces tightly in plastic. Garnish with the citrus juice just before eating.

Spicy Tangerines

Preparation time: about 5 minutes
Marinating time: several hours
Portions: 6
Calories per portion: 40

1 tablespoon honey	**6 whole allspice**
2 cups water	**5 cloves**
2 1-inch cinnamon sticks	**1 pound tangerines**

Combine all of the ingredients except the tangerines in a 2-quart nonaluminum saucepan. Place over high heat and stir to dissolve the honey. Heat to the boiling point, then boil for 1 minute.

Meanwhile, peel the tangerines. Separate the segments and re- move and discard the white membrane between them.

After the spice mixture has boiled for 1 minute, turn off the heat and remove any scum that has risen to the surface. Place the tangerines in the pan and cool to room temperature. Place in a covered container and refrigerate for several hours or overnight. To serve, remove the tangerines with a slotted spoon and discard the spices and poaching liquid.

Blueberry Pineapple Compote

Preparation time: about 5 minutes
Marinating time: 30 minutes
Portions: 3
Calories per portion: 48

4 ounces fresh pineapple chunks	**4 ounces blueberries**
	1 tablespoon 80-proof rum

Cut the pineapple into small chunks and place in a bowl with the blueberries. Pour the rum over the fruit and cover. Let the fruit marinate for 30 minutes, tossing occasionally. The fruit can be eaten right away or refrigerated. If refrigerated, remove the fruit and let sit at room temperature for 15 minutes before eating.

Creamy Grapefruit Salad

Preparation time: about 5 minutes
Portions: 1
Calories per portion: 54

1 ounce leaf lettuce
3½ ounces grapefruit sections
      and juice (from an 8-ounce
      grapefruit half)

DRESSING

1 tablespoon Fromage Blanc
      (see Index)
¼ teaspoon poppy seeds

Wash and dry the lettuce leaves. Arrange on a plate.

With a grapefruit knife, score between each section and around the outside of the fruit. Remove the sections with a spoon and place on the lettuce.

Squeeze out as much juice as possible from any fruit left in the shell. Mix the juice with the Fromage Blanc and pour over the fruit and lettuce. Garnish with the poppy seeds and eat right away.

Nectarines in Delectable Whipped Dairy Topping

This recipe for Delectable Whipped Dairy Topping is something to shout about. Thanks to the powerful blade action of the food processor, skim milk and ice cubes can be combined to produce a gorgeous, fluffy topping that looks exactly like real whipped cream and has a true dairy taste from the skim milk. It is so quickly prepared that I recommend always making it just before eating. If it is refrigerated with the optional stabilizer, it loses the beautiful soft consistency of real whipped cream.

Preparation time: about 5 minutes
Portions: 4
Calories per portion: 63

**12 ounces nectarines (2 6-
    ounce nectarines)**

DELECTABLE WHIPPED DAIRY
TOPPING

**½ cup skim milk
1 ice cube (1″ × 1″ × ¾″)**

Optional Stabilizer

**1 teaspoon unflavored gelatin
¼ cup cold water**

Wash the nectarines and dry. Cut in half and remove the pits. Slice thin. Place the fruit in four shallow fruit bowls or plates.

Place the cold milk in the food processor. Turn the machine on and add the ice cube through the feed tube. Process until the milk is very thick and looks like whipped cream (about 50–60 seconds). Spoon over the nectarines and eat right away.

To stabilize the whipped topping: Sprinkle the gelatin over the cold water in a small heatproof cup. Place the cup in a small pan of hot water and let it sit, double boiler style, until the gelatin melts (about 4–5 minutes). While processing the milk and ice, add the gelatin in a thin stream through the feed tube.

This Delectable Whipped Dairy Topping has about *52 calories* compared with a whopping *419 calories* for a comparable amount of whipped cream. Five tablespoons of the Delectable Whipped Dairy Topping will add *9 calories* to a dessert portion.

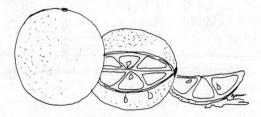

Melon Medley

Preparation time: about 10 minutes
Portions: 6
Calories per portion: 42

6 ounces cantaloupe
6 ounces honeydew

6 ounces watermelon
¼ cup dry white wine

GARNISH

Fresh mint leaves

Using a small melon baller, scoop out 6 ounces of each melon. Place in a large bowl. Pour the wine over the melon and toss. Serve right away in glass bowls, garnished with mint leaves.

COOKED FRUIT SNACKS

Hot Grapefruit with Honey and Nutmeg

This is an excellent brunch appetizer.

Preparation time: about 7 minutes
Portions: 2
Calories per portion: 48

1 13-ounce grapefruit
1 teaspoon honey
Freshly grated nutmeg

Halve the grapefruit and cut around the sections with a grapefruit knife. Remove the tough membrane and discard. Drizzle each half with ½ teaspoon of the honey and sprinkle lightly with freshly grated nutmeg. Broil for 5–7 minutes until the rind is lightly browned. Eat right away.

Baked Stuffed Peaches

Preparation time: about 5 minutes
Baking time: 45 minutes
Portions: 2
Calories per portion: 78

1 7-ounce peach
1 teaspoon finely grated lemon
   zest
¼ ounce dry bread crumbs (see
   Artichoke Stuffed with
   Ham and Cheese in Index
   for making bread crumbs)

¼ teaspoon combined freshly
   grated cinnamon and
   nutmeg
1 teaspoon unsalted butter at
   room temperature
1 teaspoon honey

Wash and dry the peach. Cut it in half through the slight indentation line that appears on the outside of the peach. Remove the pit and discard. Scoop away the thin red membrane from the pit holes.
   Preheat the oven to 375° F.
   Finely chop the lemon zest and in a small bowl combine it with the bread crumbs, spices, butter, and honey. Stuff half of the mixture into each peach half. Wrap the peaches tightly in heavy aluminum foil and place in a small, shallow baking dish. Bake for 40 minutes.
   The peaches can be eaten hot or lukewarm. Or they can be refrigerated and brought to room temperature before eating.

Chunky Applesauce

Preparation time: about 12 minutes
Portions: 3
Calories per portion: 67

13 ounces Jonathan or
   McIntosh apples
¼ cup water

⅛ teaspoon combined cloves,
   allspice, cinnamon, and
   nutmeg

Wash the apples and cut into quarters but do not peel. Remove the cores and cut each quarter into several chunks. Put the apple chunks into a small saucepan with the water. Cover and cook at a low–medium simmer until the apples are tender (about 10 minutes). Remove the lid and cook over high heat for 1 minute to cook off excess water. Press the apples with the back of a large spoon to break into chunks. Grind the spices and mix with the apples. The applesauce can be eaten hot, warm, or at room temperature.

Smooth Applesauce

Preparation time: about 15 minutes
Portions: 2
Calories per portion: 87

13 ounces Jonathan or McIntosh apples
¼ cup water

⅛ teaspoon combined cloves, allspice, cinnamon, and nutmeg

Wash the apples and cut into quarters but do not peel. Remove the cores and cut the quarters into chunks. Place in a saucepan with ¼ cup water and cook as for Chunky Applesauce. When the apples are tender, force through a sieve or the fine disc of a food mill. Season with the spices and eat hot, warm, or at room temperature.

Pears Poached in Red Wine

Preparation time: 2 minutes
Poaching time: about 20 minutes
Portions: 4
Calories per portion: 47

12 ounces Bosc pears (2 6-ounce pears), ripe but still firm
½ cup dry red wine

2 cloves
1-inch cinnamon stick
1 ½-inch vanilla bean

Wash and peel the pears and place in a small saucepan. Cover with the wine and enough cold water to cover the pears. Add the spices and cover the pan. Place over medium-high heat. When the water comes to the boil, reduce to a very low simmer. Poach the pears until very tender when pierced with a sharp knife (15–20 minutes). Cool the pears in the poaching liquid, then cut each pear in half. Remove from liquid to serve warm or at room temperature.

The pears will keep in the poaching liquid in a jar, and can be refrigerated for several weeks. The poaching liquid can be strained and reused.

Banana Sauté

This fruit snack is sure to please as a dessert or side dish for Sunday brunch.

Preparation time: about 5 minutes
Portions: 4
Calories per portion: 72

¼ cup freshly squeezed orange juice
1 teaspoon lemon juice
1 teaspoon orange zest
1 tablespoon honey

1 teaspoon unsalted butter
1 8-ounce banana, ripe but still firm
Freshly grated nutmeg

Squeeze the citrus juices and chop the orange zest. Mix with the honey and set aside.

Melt the butter in a heavy 10-inch skillet. Peel the banana. Cut it in half lengthwise, then into 4 pieces. Place the banana in the skillet and sauté over medium-high heat until the bottom side is browned (about 1 minute). Turn and sauté the other side until brown (about 1 minute).

Turn the heat up to high and add the juice and honey mixture. Cook for about 1½ minutes until a glaze forms. Remove from the heat and dust the bananas lightly with nutmeg. Serve each portion on a small plate garnished with the sauce.

Stewed Plums

Preparation time: about 10 minutes
Portions: 6
Calories per portion: 68

½ cup water
2 tablespoons honey
½ lemon

1 2-inch cinnamon stick
1 pound fresh ripe plums

Heat the water and honey until the honey dissolves and the water starts to boil. Squeeze the lemon juice into the water and then drop the lemon half into the water. Put the cinnamon stick in the water.

Wash the plums and halve them. Remove and discard the pits. Place the plums in the hot poaching liquid. Simmer for 6–8 minutes. Remove from the heat and cool to lukewarm. The plums can be eaten warm or at room temperature. Discard the cinnamon stick and lemon before eating.

Rhubarb and Strawberry Puree

Preparation time: about 20 minutes
Portions: 4
Calories per portion: 62

8 ounces rhubarb stalks,
    trimmed of leaves

8 ounces hulled strawberries
2 tablespoons honey

Wash the rhubarb and trim the ends. Cut into small chunks. Wash the berries and slice in half. Place with the rhubarb chunks in a small saucepan and put about 1 inch of water in the pan. Simmer over medium-low heat until tender (15–20 minutes). Stir the honey into the fruit and mash the fruit with the back of a spoon to make a pureelike consistency. The puree can be eaten warm or at room temperature.

Quince Compote

This rounded, greenish yellow fruit looks like a large green delicious apple, but its hard flesh must be cooked to be edible. The
cooked quince has a wonderful flavor and aroma reminiscent of
raspberries and apples. This compote makes a tasty, unusual garnish
for lamb or pork.

Preparation time: about 15 minutes
Portions: 2
Calories per portion: 87

1 8½-ounce quince   **2 teaspoons grapefruit zest**
2 tablespoons freshly squeezed   **1 tablespoon honey**
grapefruit juice

Peel and quarter the quince. Remove the seeds and cut each
quarter in half, then into 4 chunks. Place the quince chunks in a
small saucepan and place about ½ inch of water in the pan. Cover
and set over high heat until the water is hot. Reduce the heat to
medium-low and cook until the quince is tender (about 10 minutes).

Squeeze the grapefruit juice. With a citrus zester remove 2 tablespoons of zest in long thin strips. Mix the juice and zest with the
honey.

Remove the lid from the quince pan. Turn the heat up and cook
off any remaining water, tossing occasionally so the fruit does not
scorch. Add the grapefruit juice, zest, and honey to the pan. Cook
until the juice comes to a boil. Remove from the heat. The compote
can be eaten hot, warm, or at room temperature. It can also be
refrigerated and gently reheated.

4

Satisfying Soup Snacks

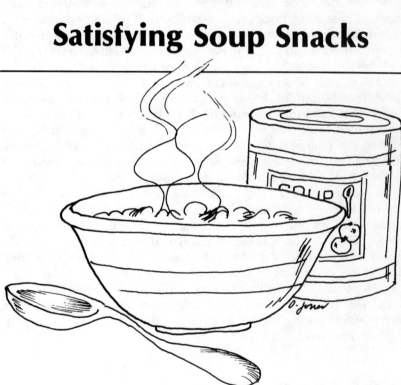

Soups are especially satisfying as slim snacks. Soups are a comforting kind of food and are good for you. When prepared with rich homemade stocks, as these soups are, they are truly sustaining. Most soups keep so well in the refrigerator or freezer that there is no excuse for not having a soup snack on hand when the hunger bell sounds.

Homemade stocks are indispensable for these satisfying soup snacks. Three basic stock recipes—chicken, fish, and vegetable—are included. Because many of the slim snacks protein recipes revolve around chicken and fish, it makes good sense to use the scraps (fish and chicken bones, etc.) to yield delicious benefits.

Stock making is neither difficult nor time-consuming in the literal sense. It does require the cook's presence while the stock simmers, but it does not require close attention. It can be made effortlessly on a stay-at-home day while other tasks are being performed. It is wise to make large batches to freeze in containers of various sizes. Hot chicken, fish, or vegetable stock, with just the addition of freshly chopped herbs, makes a delicious pick-me-up.

There are two added benefits to making homemade stock. The fat can be removed completely by chilling the stock before using, thus cutting the calorie count appreciably. And, unlike commercial stocks, which are heavily salted, homemade stock can be made salt-free. I never salt stock until the final preparation, whether it is soup or a sauce, so I maintain control of how much is added. For those who must watch their salt intake, it can be left out entirely.

These satisfying soup snacks include hot soups, well suited for fall and winter snacking, and cool refreshing soups to soothe on scorching summer days.

BASIC SOUP STOCKS

Homemade Chicken Stock

Preparation time: about 15 minutes
Cooking time: about 5 hours
Yield: 5 quarts
Calories per 1-cup portion: 44

1 5-pound stewing chicken
1 pound chicken necks, wings,
　carcasses
Cold water
4 ounces leek, trimmed of root
　end
5 ounces carrot, trimmed of
　stem end

5 ounces celery
4 ounces yellow onion,
　trimmed of root end and
　dirty outer leaves
2 cloves garlic

BOUQUET GARNI

1 ounce parsley stems
½ ounce fresh thyme or 2
　teaspoons dried
2 bay leaves

Remove the leg and breast portion from the chicken or have the butcher do it. Break the carcass in half. Place the chicken carcass and pieces in a 12-quart stockpot. Cover with cold water. Place over medium-high heat. When the water almost reaches the boil, reduce the heat. Occasionally skim any foam that rises to the top of the water.

Scrub the vegetables, but don't peel them. To clean the leek, make a slit starting 3 inches into the white part and running down through the green stem. Turn the leek 90 degrees and make another slit directly perpendicular to the first one. Leeks are usually very dirty and need to be washed thoroughly in cold water. Chop all the vegetables coarsely. Don't peel the garlic, but crush it with the blade of a heavy chef's knife.

Make a *bouquet garni* with the herbs (see technique in Chapter 1).

When the chicken and bones stop throwing scum (about 1 hour) add the chopped vegetables and *bouquet garni* to the pot. Cover with warm water, if necessary to bring the water level to the top of the vegetables. Half cover the stockpot with a lid and allow to simmer gently. Don't cover the pot completely or allow the stock to boil, or it will become cloudy. Skim the stock occasionally of any scum or pools of fat that rise to the surface.

After 3 hours, remove the leg and breast portions of the stewing chicken and place on a platter. As soon as they are cool enough to handle, use your hand to remove the meat from the bones. Remove the skin and gristle and discard. Put the bones back into the stock-pot and cook the stock for 1 hour more. When the chicken meat is completely cool, wrap in foil or plastic and refrigerate for use in another recipe. (See Index for other recipes using chicken meat.)

To strain the stock: Set a colander on top of a large bowl or pan. Line the colander with a thin cotton towel that has been rinsed several times in hot water and wrung dry. Pour or ladle the broth through the colander. Dump the bones and vegetables into the colander and allow to drain for a few minutes. Squeeze gently on the bones to remove as much stock as possible. Discard the vegetables and bones. Pour the broth into a tall container and cool at room temperature. Refrigerate the stock, uncovered, for several hours or until the fat is solidified on top. Remove the fat and discard. The stock can now be used in recipes. It will keep in the refrigerator for up to a week. If refrigerating for longer than a week, boil the stock, cool to room temperature, and then refrigerate.

To freeze the stock: Pour into plastic containers of the desired size, cover and label and freeze or line a container with a heavy plastic freezer bag, pour in the stock, cover, and freeze. When frozen, pop the bag out, seal with a twist tie, label, and put back in the freezer. For some of the *Slim Snacks* recipes that call for a small amount of stock, it may be convenient to freeze stock in an ice cube tray, then store the frozen cubes in a heavy plastic freezer bag. The stock can be thawed in the refrigerator or put frozen into a covered pan and heated.

Individual Chicken Stock Snack

Calories per 1-cup portion: 44

Freeze chicken stock in 8-ounce containers for individual chicken stock snacks. The frozen stock can be removed from the freezer and heated in a covered pan in just a few minutes. If desired, season with a pinch of kosher salt and a sprinkling of fresh chopped herb.

Fish Stock

Preparation time: about 10 minutes
Cooking time: about 3 hours
Yield: 2½ quarts
Calories per 1-cup portion: 35

2½ **pounds bones and heads from nonoily fish like turbot, red snapper, or halibut**
3 **ounces celery**
3 **ounces carrots, trimmed of stem end**

3 **ounces yellow onion, root end and dirty outer leaves removed**
3 **ounces leek, trimmed of root end**
1 **cup dry white wine**
About 2 quarts cold water

BOUQUET GARNI

1 **ounce parsley stems**
¼ **ounce fresh thyme or 1 teaspoon dried**

1 **bay leaf**
3–4 **white peppercorns**

Wash the fish bones thoroughly in cold water, using a small knife to slit the membrane along the backbone, which holds blood. Remove the gills (the reddish, fan-shaped sections on each side of the head) with a sharp knife or scissors. Rinse thoroughly (any blood left along the bones will make a muddy stock).

Place the bones in a 6-quart nonaluminum pot. Scrub the vegetables but don't peel. (See preceding recipe for leek-cleaning technique.) Chop the vegetables coarsely and put in the pot with the fish bones. Add the wine and enough cold water to cover. Make the *bouquet garni* (see technique in Chapter 1) and place in the pot.

Heat the mixture until almost boiling, then reduce to a simmer. Skim any foam that rises to the surface. Simmer the bones and vegetables, partially covered, for about 3 hours, skimming when necessary. If the liquid falls below the solids in the pot, add warm water to just cover the solids. Strain and cool according to the directions in the preceding recipe.

The fish stock can be refrigerated for up to 2 days. If storing longer in the refrigerator, boil, cool, and refrigerate again to prevent spoilage. The fish stock can be frozen for use in sauces, in poaching fish, or in soups.

Individual Fish Stock Snack

Calories per 1-cup portion: 35

Freeze the fish stock in 8-ounce containers for individual fish stock snacks. The frozen stock can be removed from the freezer and heated in a covered pan in just a few minutes. If desired, season with a pinch of kosher salt and a sprinkling of fresh chopped herb.

Homemade Vegetable Stock

Preparation time: 10 minutes
Cooking time: 2 hours
Yield: 2 quarts
Calories per 1-cup portion: 25

**5 ounces carrots, trimmed of
 stem end**
5 ounces celery
4 ounces turnip
**12 ounces leek, trimmed of
 root end**

**8 ounces yellow onion,
 trimmed of root end and
 dirty outer leaves**
2 cloves garlic

BOUQUET GARNI

½ ounce parsley stems
**¼ ounce fresh thyme or 1
 teaspoon dried**
1 bay leaf

Scrub the carrots, celery, and turnip but don't peel. See leek-cleaning technique in Homemade Chicken Stock. Chop the vegetables coarsely. Slice the onion into ½-inch slices and smash the garlic with the blade of a heavy chef's knife. Prepare the *bouquet garni* according to the instructions in Chapter 1.

Place all the vegetables and the *bouquet garni* in a 6-quart pot. Cover with cold water and heat over medium-high heat. Just before the mixture comes to a boil, reduce the heat to a gentle simmer. Cook for 2 hours. Skim any foam that rises to the surface. Keep the pot three-quarters covered with a lid.

After 2 hours, strain the stock through a colander lined with a thin cotton towel that has been well rinsed in hot water and wrung dry. The stock can be stored in the refrigerator for up to a week. If storing longer in the refrigerator, reboil the stock after 1 week, cool, and refrigerate again to prevent spoilage.

Individual Vegetable Stock Snack

Calories per 1-cup portion: 25

Freeze the vegetable stock in 8-ounce containers. For a quick snack, pop a frozen cup of vegetable stock into a small saucepan. Cook, covered, until the broth boils. If desired, season with a pinch of kosher salt and a sprinkling of fresh chopped herb.

HOT VEGETABLE SOUPS

Creamy Cauliflower and Tarragon Soup

Preparation time: about 20 minutes
Portions: 4
Calories per portion: 64

1 cup Homemade Chicken
   Stock (see Index)
3 ounces potatoes
1 ounce yellow onion
12 ounces cauliflower flowerets

2 teaspoons fresh or frozen
   tarragon leaves
¾ cup skim milk
¼ teaspoon kosher salt
Pinch of white pepper

Heat the chicken stock in a 1-quart saucepan.

Peel the potatoes and onion and chop into small pieces. Add to the stock and cover. Simmer over medium heat for 10 minutes.

Trim the core from the cauliflower and weigh 12 ounces of

flowerets. Chop them into small pieces. Add the cauliflower to the stock and cook, covered, until tender (6–8 minutes). Chop the tarragon and set aside.

Remove the vegetables from the stock and puree in a blender or food processor fitted with the steel blade or through a food mill. Mix the puree with the stock and return to medium heat. Add the skim milk, chopped tarragon, and pepper and salt. The soup can be eaten right away or cooled, refrigerated, and gently reheated.

Lentil Soup

Preparation time: about 40 minutes
Portions: 10
Calories per portion: 72

4 small cloves garlic or 2 large ones
6 ounces green lentils

1½ cups Homemade Chicken Stock (see Index)
2 cups water

BOUQUET GARNI

¼ ounce parsley stems
⅛ ounce fresh thyme leaves or ½ teaspoon dried
1 small bay leaf

---

2 ounces celery
2 ounces carrot, trimmed of stem end

2 ounces yellow onion
Freshly ground black pepper
½ teaspoon kosher salt

GARNISH

1 tablespoon Italian parsley leaves

Mince the garlic. Combine with the lentils in a 4-quart pan along with the stock and water. Prepare the *bouquet garni* according to the instructions in Chapter 1. Place the *bouquet garni* in the pan, cover, and place over high heat. When the liquid boils, reduce the heat right away and simmer gently for 25 minutes.

Chop the remaining vegetables very fine. Chop the parsley and set aside. After the lentils have cooked 25 minutes, add the chopped vegetables to the pan and cook for 15 minutes more. Remove from the heat and puree 1 cup of the lentils in a blender or a food processor fitted with the steel blade or through a food mill. Mix the puree with the cooked lentils. Season with freshly ground black pepper and salt. The soup can be eaten right away or cooled, refrigerated, and reheated. Serve with the freshly chopped parsley as a garnish.

Fresh Tomato Puree

Preparation time: about 20 minutes
Portions: 4
Calories per portion: 35

**14 ounces fresh ripe tomatoes
or 1 28-ounce can
tomatoes**
**2 teaspoons fresh or frozen
basil leaves**

⅔ cup skim milk
Pinch of kosher salt
Freshly ground black pepper

If using fresh tomatoes, remove the core, skin, and seeds. If using canned tomatoes, remove the seeds and strain the juice to save for another recipe. (See both techniques in Ratatouille.)

Chop the tomatoes coarsely and place in a small heavy saucepan. Cover and cook at a gentle simmer for 15 minutes.

Roll the basil leaves into a tight bundle and cut into thin slices. Set aside. Puree the cooked tomatoes in a blender or food processor fitted with the steel blade or through a food mill. Return the puree to the pan and add the milk. Gently heat the soup and season with salt and pepper. Serve garnished with the basil. If making the soup in advance, reheat gently and chop the basil just before serving.

Potato Onion Soup

Preparation time: about 22 minutes
Portions: 2
Calories per portion: 74

4 ounces red potatoes
1½ ounces yellow onion
½ cup skim milk
¼ teaspoon kosher salt

Freshly ground black pepper
½ teaspoon Italian parsley
   leaves or fresh cilantro
   leaves

Scrub the potatoes. If small, cut in half and then into thin slices. If the potatoes are fairly large, cut into quarters, then into thin slices. Peel the onion and slice thin. Put the onions and potatoes into a small saucepan. Cover with the milk. Add the salt. Cover and bring almost to a boil. Reduce to a simmer and leave the lid slightly ajar so the milk does not boil over. Cook until the potatoes are tender (about 20 minutes). Chop the herb. Season the soup with freshly ground black pepper and the chopped herb. If desired, puree about ⅓ of the potatoes and onions and mix with the remaining soup to make it thicker.

Broccoli Puree

Preparation time: about 20 minutes
Portions: 4
Calories per portion: 67

1 cup Homemade Chicken
   Stock (see Index)
3 ounces potatoes
12 ounces broccoli flowerets

¾ cup skim milk
½ teaspoon kosher salt
Pinch of white pepper

Heat the chicken stock in a 1-quart saucepan. Peel the potatoes and cut into small cubes. Add the potatoes to the stock and cover. Simmer over medium heat for 10 minutes.

Trim and peel the broccoli. Chop into small pieces. Add the broccoli to the potatoes and stock and cook until tender (6–8 minutes). Remove the vegetables from the stock and puree in a blender or food processor fitted with the steel blade or through a food mill.

Mix the puree with the stock and return to medium heat. Add the skim milk and season with salt and pepper. The soup can be eaten right away or cooled, refrigerated, and gently reheated.

French Onion Soup

Preparation time: about 35 minutes
Portions: 4
Calories per portion: 99

6 ounces yellow onion
1 tablespoon water or more
2½ cups Homemade Chicken
   Stock (see Index)
¼ teaspoon kosher salt
Freshly ground black pepper
1 ounce Gruyère cheese

1 ounce French bread, cut into
   4 slices
1 garlic clove
1 tablespoon grated imported
   Parmesan cheese, very
   loosely packed

Preheat the oven to 400° F.

Peel the onions and slice. Place them in a heavy sauté pan with 1 tablespoon of water. Cover for 5 minutes and place over medium heat until onions start to exude their moisture. Uncover and turn up the heat to medium-high. Toss the onions frequently until they are very soft and golden in color. If they begin to brown too much, add 1–2 more tablespoons of water to the pan. Add the stock to the pan to heat. Season with salt and pepper.

Shred the Gruyère cheese on the coarse side of a cheese grater. Set aside. Toast the bread slices on each side and while still warm rub with the halved garlic clove. Discard the garlic. Place one piece of bread in each bottom of 4 1-cup ovenproof ramekins or bowls. Ladle equal amounts of the onion broth into each ramekin. Sprinkle the Parmesan evenly over the four bowls, then sprinkle with the Gruyère. Place the ramekins on a baking sheet and bake in the oven until the cheese is lightly browned and bubbly (about 20 minutes). Remove from the oven and allow to sit for a few minutes before eating.

Dill-icious Carrot Soup

Preparation time: about 20 minutes
Portions: 4
Calories per portion: 68

8 ounces carrots, trimmed of
    stem ends
1½ cups skim milk
⅛ teaspoon dried dill seed

¼ teaspoon kosher salt
½ cup Slim Snacks Yogurt (see
    Index)

GARNISH

1 teaspoon chopped Italian
    parsley or fresh dill

Fill a 4-quart saucepan with about 2 inches of water. Cover and set on high heat. Scrub the carrots and cut into ½-inch circles. When the water comes to a boil, place an adjustable, nonaluminum steamer rack into the pan. Place the carrots on the rack, cover the pan, and bring back to the boil. Reduce to a simmer and steam until the carrots are tender (about 15 minutes).

Puree the carrots in a blender or food processor fitted with a steel blade or through the fine disc of a food mill. Place the puree in a saucepan. Add the milk to the pan. Coarsely crush the dill seeds with the mortar and pestle and add to the pan. Heat gently for about 5 minutes. Add the salt.

Remove the soup from the heat and gently stir in the yogurt. Garnish with the chopped parsley or dill and eat right away.

Celery Soup

Preparation time: about 30 minutes
Portions: 4
Calories per portion: 37

8 ounces celery
2 ounces yellow onion
1 cup Homemade Chicken
    Stock (see Index)

⅛ teaspoon cumin seeds
½ cup skim milk
¼ teaspoon kosher salt

Scrub the celery and remove the tough strings. Chop into ½-inch pieces. Peel the onion and chop coarse. Place the vegetables in a 1-quart saucepan with the chicken stock. Grind the cumin seeds in a spice grinder or with a mortar and pestle and add to the vegetables. Cover and bring to a boil. Reduce the heat and cook, covered, until the celery is tender (about 25 minutes).

With a slotted spoon or skimmer, transfer the celery and onion to a food processor fitted with a steel blade, a food mill, or a blender. Puree the celery and onion. Return the puree to the pan with the stock. Add the milk and salt. Heat gently. Serve right away or cool, refrigerate, and gently reheat.

Wild Mushroom Soup

European wild mushrooms (*Boletus edulis*) are available dried in many supermarkets and gourmet food shops. The incredibly rich broth from reconstituted wild mushrooms can add gusto to winter soups, meats, and vegetable dishes.

Preparation time: about 15 minutes
Soaking time: 30 minutes
Portions: 4
Calories per portion: 44

½ ounce dried European
    mushrooms (such as
    porcini or cepès)
8 ounces fresh white
    mushrooms
½ teaspoon fresh or frozen
    thyme leaves or ⅛
    teaspoon dried

1 teaspoon unsalted butter
1½ cups Homemade Chicken
    Stock (see Index)
⅛ teaspoon kosher salt
Freshly ground black pepper

Put the dried mushrooms into a small cup with ½ cup warm water. Set aside to soak for 30 minutes.

Clean the fresh mushrooms with a mushroom brush or damp cloth. Cut off the ends and slice the mushrooms. Chop the thyme.

Melt the butter in a 10-inch sauté pan. Coat the bottom of the pan with the melted butter, then add the fresh mushrooms. Sprinkle the thyme over the mushrooms and cover with a heavy lid. Cook over medium heat for 1–2 minutes, until the mushrooms start to exude moisture. Remove the lid and turn the heat up to high. Toss the mushrooms for 3–4 minutes.

Drain the wild mushrooms through a fine sieve lined with cheesecloth or a paper towel. Reserve liquid. Place the mushrooms in the sieve and rinse quickly under cold water. Chop the wild mushrooms very fine and add to the pan with the fresh mushrooms. Add the mushroom liquid and chicken stock to the pan. Simmer, covered, for 10 minutes. Season with salt and pepper. Eat right away or cool, refrigerate, and gently reheat.

Pumpkin Soup

Preparation time: about 12 minutes
Portions: 2
Calories per portion: 69

1 ounce yellow onion
½ cup Pumpkin Puree (see Index)
1 cup skim milk
1½ teaspoons fresh marjoram leaves or ½ teaspoon dried
¼ teaspoon kosher salt

Chop the onion very fine and place in a small saucepan with the pumpkin puree and the milk. If using dried marjoram, crush the leaves in a mortar and pestle. If using fresh marjoram, chop the leaves fine. Add the marjoram and salt to the pan. Cover and simmer gently over medium heat for 10 minutes. Eat right away or cool, refrigerate, and gently reheat. If using dried marjoram, garnish with some fresh Italian parsley.

Japanese Tofu Soup

Tofu, pressed soybean curd, is an excellent low-fat source of protein. It is available in Oriental food stores and in supermarkets in many urban areas.

Preparation time: about 5 minutes
Portions: 4
Calories per portion: 75

3 cups Homemade Chicken
   Stock (see Index)
3 ounces fresh spinach leaves,
   trimmed of spines and
   stems
1 ounce scallion, trimmed of
   root end

¼ teaspoon kosher salt
½ tablespoon imported
   Japanese soy sauce or ¼
   tablespoon Chinese soy
   sauce
6 ounces tofu
¾ teaspoon gingerroot

Put the chicken stock into a 2-quart saucepan and cover. Place over high heat.

Wash the spinach leaves and remove the tough stems and spines. Weigh 3 ounces of cleaned leaves. Cut the spinach into thin strips. Wash the scallion and slice into thin circles.

When the stock boils, add the scallion, spinach, salt, and soy sauce. Reduce the heat to medium-low and simmer for 3–4 minutes.

Cut the tofu into small cubes and finely chop or grate the gingerroot. Add these ingredients to the soup and heat for 1 minute. Eat right away or cool, refrigerate, and gently reheat.

HOT FISH AND CHICKEN SOUPS

Clam Chowder

Preparation time: about 30 minutes (less time if using canned
   clams)
Portions: 6
Calories per portion: 65

5 ounces of shucked clams with
   their liquor (approximately
   1 quart of clams in the
   shell; because clams vary
   in size, check with the fish
   merchant about how many
   clams are needed to yield
   5 ounces) or 1 10-ounce
   can baby clams
1 teaspoon unsalted butter
2 ounces yellow onion

6 ounces red potato
⅔ cup clam liquor from the
   shelled clams (use Fish
   Stock to make ⅔ cup if
   there is not enough liquor;
   see Index)
1 cup skim milk
1 tablespoon chopped Italian
   parsley leaves
Pinch of kosher salt, if needed
Freshly ground black pepper

If using clams in the shells, scrub the shells well under cold water. Place a fine sieve over a bowl and open the clams over the bowl to catch the liquor. Insert the tip of a clam knife or other strong thin knife between the two shells. Cut the muscle at the hinged back of the clam. Open the shell and remove the clam. Pour any remaining liquor into the bowl. Repeat until all the clams are shucked. Set the clams aside. If using canned clams or clams that have already been shucked, drain the liquor from the clams and set aside.

In a small skillet, melt the butter. Peel the onion and slice thin. Place the onion in the pan with the butter and stew for about 5 minutes. If the onion starts to brown, add a spoonful of water to the pan. Peel the potato and cut into small chunks. Place in a 2-quart saucepan with the clam liquor and milk. Add the onion to the saucepan. Simmer, partially covered, for about 15–20 minutes. Skim foam from the top when necessary. Chop the parsley and set aside.

When the potatoes are tender, use the back of a large spoon to smash them against the side of the pan. Add the clams to the chowder and heat the clams (2–3 minutes). Canned clams will need no extra salt, but the fresh clams may need a pinch of kosher salt. Add 3–4 grinds of black pepper to the pan and stir. Serve right away, garnished with the chopped parsley. If making the chowder in advance, cool, refrigerate, and gently reheat. Garnish with the parsley just before eating.

Catch-of-the-Day Soup

Preparation time: about 15 minutes
Portions: 6
Calories per portion: 61

2 cups Fish Stock (see Index)
¼ teaspoon kosher salt
2 ounces red potato
2 ounces carrot, trimmed of
    stem end
2 ounces shelled fresh peas or
    2 ounces frozen peas
2 ounces yellow onion

1 tablespoon fresh cilantro or
    fennel leaves
6 ounces firm-fleshed, nonoily
    white fish such as red
    snapper, flounder, turbot,
    halibut, trimmed of bones
    and skin

Put the fish stock and salt into a 2-quart saucepan. Cover and place over high heat.

Scrub the potato and carrot. Cut the potato into cubes. Cut the carrot into small chunks. If using fresh peas, shell the peas and weigh 2 ounces. Chop the onion medium-fine. Chop the herb and set aside.

When the stock boils, reduce the heat and add the potatoes and carrots to the pan. Cook partially covered for 10 minutes. Skim any foam that rises to the top of the stock. Add the peas and onion to the stock and cook for 5 minutes more.

Cut the fish into small chunks. Add to the pan and cook for 3 minutes. If using cooked fish left over from making fish stock, chill the fish, then pick the flesh from the bones. Weigh the fish, then supplement with uncooked fish fillets, if necessary, to make 6 ounces. Add the cooked fish to the soup at the last minute and cook until just heated through. Serve right away garnished with chopped cilantro or fennel.

Hearty Chicken Vegetable Soup

Preparation time: about 35 minutes
Portions: 10
Calories per portion: 66

4 ounces carrots, trimmed of stem end
5 ounces celery
7 ounces red potatoes
4 ounces yellow onion
1 quart Homemade Chicken Stock (see Index)
½ teaspoon kosher salt

5 ounces fresh or canned tomatoes
4 ounces cooked chicken, half dark and half white meat (use chicken left over from making chicken stock or from plain roast chicken)

Scrub the vegetables. Cut the carrots and celery into small pieces. Cut the potatoes into small cubes. Peel the onion and cut into small pieces. Put the vegetables into a 4-quart saucepan and cover with the chicken stock. Add the salt. Cover and place over high heat. When the stock boils, reduce the heat to a simmer. Cook until the vegetables are tender (about 20 minutes).

Core the tomato and cut in half. Gently squeeze out the seeds. If using canned tomatoes, remove the seeds. Chop the tomato into small pieces. Cut the chicken into chunks, cutting across the grain of the meat.

Add the tomato and chicken to the soup and cook for 5 minutes. The soup can be eaten right away or cooled, refrigerated, and reheated.

Bok Choy Chicken Soup

Preparation time: about 15 minutes
Portions: 10
Calories per portion: 58

2¼ ounces raw rice (enriched or parboiled)
1 quart Homemade Chicken Stock (see Index)
9-ounce head of bok choy
3 ounces scallion, white and green part, trimmed of root end

3 ounces skinned and boned chicken breast, raw
1½ ounces Fresh Bean Sprouts (see Index)
½ teaspoon kosher salt
Generous pinch of white pepper

Place the rice and stock in a 4-quart saucepan. Cover and place over high heat. When stock boils, reduce the heat and simmer for 10 minutes.

Wash the bok choy and cut into thin diagonal slices. Set aside. Cut the scallion into thin diagonal slices. Set aside. Cut the chicken into thin strips across the grain. Place the chicken strips with the scallions.

After cooking the rice for 10 minutes, add the bok choy to the pan. Cover and cook over medium-high heat for 2 minutes. Add the scallions and chicken strips. Stir. Cover the pan and cook for 1 minute. Add the bean sprouts and stir. Cover the pan and cook for 30 seconds. Season with salt and pepper. Serve right away or cool, refrigerate, and gently reheat.

CHILLED SOUPS

Cool Avocado Soup

This soup is a beautiful first course for an elegant summer dinner.

Preparation time: about 12 minutes
Chilling time: several hours
Portions: 6
Calories per portion: 112

1½ ounces yellow onion
3 cups Homemade Chicken
 Stock (see Index)
12 ounces very ripe avocado
¼ teaspoon kosher salt

⅛ teaspoon freshly ground
 black pepper
Several dashes of cayenne
 pepper

GARNISH

4 thin lemon slices
1 teaspoon fresh cilantro

Slice the onion very thin and place in a 2-quart saucepan with the chicken stock. Cover and place over high heat. When the stock boils, reduce the heat to a simmer. Cook until the onions are tender (6–7 minutes).

Cut the avocado in half and spear the pit with a sharp knife. Discard the pit. Lift the two halves out of the shell and slice thin. Place in the stock pan. With a spoon, scrape the inside of the avocado shell to remove all the flesh. Add to the stock. Simmer for 3 minutes.

Remove the onion and avocado slices and puree in a food processor fitted with a steel blade, in a blender, or through a food mill. Put the puree and the stock in a glass or ceramic bowl. Add the seasonings and mix. Cover and refrigerate for several hours. Serve garnished with a lemon slice and freshly chopped cilantro.

Chilled Strawberry Soup

Preparation time: about 10 minutes
Chilling time: several hours
Portions: 6
Calories per portion: 90

1 quart fresh, very ripe
   strawberries (3 berries can
   be saved for garnish)
1 cup dry white wine

2½ cups naturally sparkling
   water or pure seltzer water
4 tablespoons lemon juice or
   less to taste
Freshly ground black pepper

GARNISH

3 sliced strawberries
Fresh mint leaves

Wash and hull the berries. Puree the strawberries in a food processor fitted with the steel blade, in a blender, or through a food mill. Heat the wine and simmer for 5 minutes in a nonaluminum pan. Remove the wine from the heat. Add the water, puree, lemon juice, and some freshly ground black pepper. Adjust seasoning to taste. Cover and chill for several hours. Serve in chilled glass bowls garnished with sliced strawberries and a fresh mint leaf.

Slim Vichyssoise

Preparation time: about 15 minutes
Cooking time: about 30 minutes
Chilling time: several hours
Portions: 6
Calories per portion: 74

9 ounces leek, white part only
   (the white part from about
   1 pound leek)
2 ounces yellow onion

8 ounces red potato
½ teaspoon kosher salt
2 cups skim milk

GARNISH

2 teaspoons fresh chives

Clean the leeks (see technique in Homemade Chicken Stock). Cut off the white part and reserve the green part for stock or another purpose. Slice the white part thin. Slice the yellow onion thin. Scrub the potato and peel. Cut into thin slices. Place the vegetables and salt in a 4-quart saucepan and cover with 3 cups water. Cover and place over high heat. When the water boils, reduce the heat and simmer, partially covered, for 25–30 minutes, until the vegetables are soft.

Puree the vegetables through a food mill, in a blender, or in a food processor fitted with a steel blade. Return the puree to the pan and add the milk. Heat the soup, then force it through a fine sieve to remove any fibers. Cover and refrigerate until well chilled. If soup thickens too much during chilling, thin it with ice water until it reaches the right consistency. Serve in chilled cups or bowls garnished with a sprinkle of freshly cut chives.

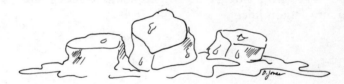

Gazpacho

Preparation time: about 20 minutes
Chilling time: several hours
Portions: 6
Calories per portion: 41

2 pounds ripe tomatoes
2 ounces green or red bell pepper, trimmed of stem, ribs, and seeds
2 ounces celery
3 ounces scallion, white and green part, trimmed of root end

3 ounces cucumbers, seeds removed (see technique in Creamy Cucumber Salad)
¼ teaspoon kosher salt
⅛ teaspoon freshly ground black pepper

Bring a 2-quart pan of water, covered, to the boil. Use the hot water to blanch the tomatoes, then remove cores, skins, and seeds according to the technique in Ratatouille. Puree the tomatoes in a food processor fitted with a steel blade or in a blender.

Chop the remaining vegetables into small pieces and combine in a glass or ceramic bowl with the tomato puree. Add seasonings and mix. Chill for several hours before eating.

Chilled Borscht with Fresh Vegetables and Dill

Preparation time: about 30 minutes
Chilling time: several hours
Portions: 4
Calories per portion: 47

8 ounces fresh beets, without green tops
1 teaspoon red wine vinegar
2 teaspoons lemon juice

1 tablespoon sugar
¾ teaspoon kosher salt
½ cup Slim Snacks Yogurt (see Index)

GARNISH

2 ounces scallion, white and green part, trimmed of root end

2 ounces cucumber, seeds removed (see technique in Creamy Cucumber Salad)
1 tablespoon fresh dill leaves
Grated beets

Scrub the beets well under cold water and leave 1 inch of stem attached to the beets. Place them in a saucepan with 2½ cups water. Bring to a boil, then reduce the heat to a rapid simmer. Let the beets cook until tender (about 20 minutes).

Scrub the garnish vegetables and cut into small pieces of equal size. Chop the fresh dill. Put the vegetables and dill in separate containers, seal well, and refrigerate.

When the beets are cooked, drain and reserve the cooking liquid. Rinse the beets under cold water and rub off the peel. Grate the beets on the coarsest side of a vegetable grater. Return ½ the beets to the cooking liquid. Reserve the other ½ for garnish. Season with vinegar, lemon juice, sugar, and salt. Add the yogurt and mix. Refrigerate until well chilled. Serve in clear glass bowls and garnish with the vegetables and chopped dill.

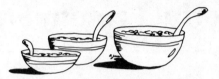

Slender Jellied Consommé

Preparation time: about 5 minutes
Chilling time: about 2 hours
Portions: 1
Calories per portion: 41

¾ cup Homemade Chicken
   Stock (see Index)
Pinch of kosher salt
⅓ ounce celery

⅓ ounce green pepper,
   trimmed of stem, ribs, and
   seeds
⅓ ounce scallion, trimmed of
   root end

GARNISH

¼ teaspoon fresh cilantro

Heat the chicken stock with the salt. Cool to room temperature. Chop the vegetables very fine. Combine. In a small glass bowl, mix ½ the vegetables with ½ the stock. Chill for 1 hour or until partially set.

Combine the remaining vegetables and stock and pour over the first ½. Cover and chill until set (can be refrigerated for several days before eating). Serve garnished with freshly chopped cilantro.

5
Powerful Protein Snacks

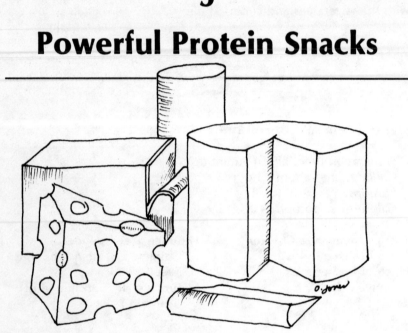

Proteins are the muscle men of the nutrition world. They are the body builders that make up and repair human tissue. Several times a day, every day, we need to replenish our protein supply from two basic food groups: the milk-cheese group and the meat-poultry-fish-beans group.

These powerful protein snacks feature proteins that are relatively low in fat, thereby lessening the total calorie intake: low-fat cheeses, skim-milk yogurt, eggs, seafood and fish, poultry, and legumes.

A small portion of a protein snack eaten at midafternoon will bridge the hunger gap between lunch and dinner. The staying power of these protein snacks will far outdistance the nutritionally empty, sugar-packed vending machine temptations.

DAIRY SNACKS

Slim Snacks Yogurt

This tangy, versatile yogurt contributes its goodness to dozens of slim snacks and makes a refreshing snack all by itself.

Preparation time: about 30 minutes
Resting time: at least 12 hours
Yield: 1 quart
Calories per cup: 88

4 cups skim milk
1 teaspoon plain commercial
    yogurt or Slim Snacks
    Yogurt

Heat the milk in a nonaluminum pan to 170–180° F. (Use a candy thermometer or an instant reading thermometer to determine the temperature.) Maintain the temperature for 3 minutes, then pour the milk into a bowl. Let the milk cool to 110 degrees, stirring occasionally to speed the cooling.

When the milk reaches 110° F., stir in the 1 teaspoon of plain yogurt. Mix well and pour into a 1-quart thermos bottle or glass jar.

Cover tightly. If using a thermos, set aside for 12 hours. If using a glass jar, set it in a spot with a steady temperature of 110° F. (for instance, a gas oven with the pilot light on) or wrap in a heavy blanket or down jacket and let it rest for 12 hours. When the yogurt thickens to the consistency of custard, it is ready to be refrigerated. The yogurt can be refrigerated for up to a week. Use as directed in individual recipes or as a snack by itself.

Slim Snacks Fruit Yogurts

These fruit yogurts taste better and fresher than the sweetened, higher-calorie commercial fruit yogurts.

Preparation time: about 2 minutes
Portions: 1

For each serving combine ¾ cup Slim Snacks Yogurt (see preceding recipe) with 2 ounces of cleaned, seeded, finely chopped fruit. Stir and enjoy.

Flavor	Calories per portion
Blueberry Yogurt	101
Strawberry Yogurt	87
Raspberry Yogurt	98
Apple Yogurt with dash of cinnamon	99
Pear Yogurt with dash of nutmeg	101
Orange Yogurt with mint	92
Peach Yogurt	88
Cantaloupe Yogurt	83
Grape Yogurt	104
Plum Yogurt	104
Banana Yogurt	114
Pineapple Yogurt	96

Yogurt Cheese

Preparation time: about 5 minutes
Draining time: 12 hours
Portions: 2
Calories per portion: 90

1 pint Slim Snacks Yogurt (see Index)

Holding up the corners of a cotton or linen kitchen towel with one hand, place the yogurt in the center of the towel. Gather the corners together and tie tightly with kitchen string. Tie the string to a sturdy wooden dowel and place over a large deep bowl or stockpot. Or tie to the kitchen faucet and let the yogurt drip into the sink overnight. Let the yogurt drain for at least 12 hours or as long as 24. Remove the cheese from the towel and refrigerate.

Fresh Yogurt Cheese with Herbs: For each serving, add ¼ teaspoon freshly chopped chives, basil, cilantro, tarragon, or mint.

Fresh Yogurt Cheese with Spices: For each serving, dust lightly with freshly ground cinnamon, nutmeg, or allspice.

Fromage Blanc (A Fresh Tart Cheese)

Preparation time: about 3 minutes
Portions: 2
Calories per portion: 54

1 ounce low-fat cottage cheese
⅓ cup Slim Snacks Yogurt (see Index)
1 teaspoon lemon juice

Place all the ingredients in a food processor fitted with a steel blade or in a blender. Process until smooth, scraping down the sides of the bowl as necessary. Serve over fresh fruit.

Fromage Blanc with Pineapple

Preparation time: about 2 minutes
Portions: 1
Calories per portion: 98

3 ounces fresh pineapple
⅓ cup Fromage Blanc (see
    preceding recipe)

Cut the pineapple into small chunks. Spoon the Fromage Blanc on top.

Fromage Blanc with Raspberries

Preparation time: about 3 minutes
Portions: 1
Calories per portion: 103

3 ounces fresh raspberries
½ cup Fromage Blanc (see
    preceding recipe)

Wash the berries. Drain well and serve in a bowl with the Fromage Blanc on top.

Zucchini Crust Quiche

This is a luscious quiche with only one-quarter the calories of the traditional Quiche Lorraine.

Preparation time: about 20 minutes
Baking time: 35 minutes
Portions: 8
Calories per portion: 120

CRUST

1½ pounds firm small zucchini
½ ounce scallion, white and
   green part, trimmed of
   root end
2 ounces shredded Gruyère
   cheese, preferably
   imported

1 tablespoon grated imported
   Parmesan cheese, very
   loosely packed
1 ounce fine dry bread crumbs
   (see technique in
   Artichoke Stuffed with
   Ham and Cheese)
1 large egg

FILLING

2 large eggs
1½ cups whole milk

½ teaspoon kosher salt
½ teaspoon freshly grated
   nutmeg

Wash the zucchini. Cut off the stem ends and the bottom tips. Shred on the coarse side of a vegetable grater. Wash the scallion and cut into 1-inch-long pieces. Cut the pieces into julienne strips. Combine with the zucchini and place in a heavy 10-inch cold sauté pan. Place the pan over high heat. When the zucchini starts to get hot on the bottom, toss with a wooden fork or spoon. Keep tossing over high heat for about 5 minutes until the zucchini is bright green and much of the moisture is evaporated. Drain in a colander and press with the back of a large spoon to squeeze out moisture. Set aside to cool for a few minutes.

Preheat the oven to 400° F.

Shred the Gruyère cheese on the coarse side of a cheese grater. Grate the Parmesan and set aside.

When the zucchini is cool enough to handle, squeeze with the hands or with paper toweling to remove as much moisture as possible. Place the zucchini in a mixing bowl and toss with the bread crumbs. In a small bowl, beat the egg, then toss with the zucchini and bread crumbs. Press the zucchini into a 9½-inch quiche pan or pie plate of nonstick material, glass, ceramic, or porcelain. Press the zucchini tightly and evenly into the plate and against the sides. The side crust should be at least ¼ inch thick. Sprinkle the cheeses over the bottom and place the quiche pan in the oven for about 10 minutes, until it starts to brown lightly.

While the crust is in the oven, beat the 2 eggs in a mixing bowl and add the milk. Season with salt and nutmeg. Set aside.

After the crust has been in the oven for 10 minutes, remove it and reduce the oven temperature to 350° F. Gently pour the filling into the crust and return the pan to the oven. Bake for about 25 minutes more, until a knife inserted in the center comes out clean. Remove the quiche from the oven and allow to set 10 minutes before cutting into wedges *or* cool the quiche and serve at room temperature *or* cool and refrigerate.

Cheesy Spinach Bundles

These cheesy spinach snacks also make a fabulous do-ahead hors d'oeuvre.

Preparation time: about 25 minutes
Portions: 20
Calories per portion: 20

20 large raw spinach leaves (3″ × 2″ or larger), weighing about 4 ounces

8 ounces part-skim ricotta cheese

2 tablespoons grated imported Parmesan cheese, very loosely packed

½ ounce scallion, white and green part, trimmed of root end

1 tablespoon lemon juice

⅛ teaspoon freshly ground black pepper

¼ teaspoon kosher salt

⅛ teaspoon freshly grated nutmeg

Wash the spinach and remove the stems. Heat 1 quart of salted water in a saucepan. When the water boils, reduce to a simmer. With a slotted spoon or large skimmer dip 2 or 3 of the spinach leaves into the water and lift out immediately. Carefully open the leaves and spread them out on paper towels, with the underside of the leaf facing up. Repeat with the remaining leaves.

If the ricotta is wet, squeeze dry (see technique in Provençal Vegetable Gratin). Grate the Parmesan and mix with the ricotta and seasonings in a bowl.

Place about ¾ tablespoon of the cheese mixture on the center of each spinach leaf. Fold the stem ends of each leaf over the cheese, then fold the sides of the leaf onto the center. Roll the cheese ball toward the top of the leaf, making a neat bundle. Repeat until all the bundles are formed. Cover and store in the refrigerator.

Neufchâtel-Sprout Sandwich

Preparation time: about 2 minutes
Portions: 1
Calories per portion: 85

½ slice Ann's Whole Wheat
    Bread (see Index)
½ ounce Neufchâtel cheese at
    room temperature

½ ounce Fresh Bean Sprouts
    (see Index)

Spread the cheese on the bread. Top with the sprouts and eat right away.

Cheddar Cheese Melt

Preparation time: about 5 minutes
Portions: 1
Calories per portion: 101

½ slice Ann's Whole Wheat
    Bread (see Index)
½-ounce slice cheddar cheese

Place the cheese on top of the whole wheat bread. Place 4 inches under the broiler flame and broil until cheese is melted and bubbly. Eat right away.

EGG SNACKS

Devilishly Good Eggs

Preparation time: about 20 minutes
Portions: 4
Calories per portion: 45

2 large eggs	**Dash of kosher salt**
¼ teaspoon coriander seeds	**Dash of freshly ground black**
1 tablespoon Slim Snacks	** pepper**
** Yogurt (see Index)**	

GARNISH

1 tablespoon Italian parsley

Bring a small pan of water to the boil. Put the eggs in the pan and cook at a gentle simmer for 10 minutes. Transfer the eggs to a bowl of cold water. Let the eggs cool.

Grind the coriander seeds in a spice grinder or with a mortar and pestle. Chop the parsley very fine and set aside.

Shell the eggs and cut in half lengthwise. Remove the yolks and mash them in a small bowl. Add the yogurt, salt, pepper, and coriander. Spoon the yolk mixture back into the white portions. Sprinkle with chopped parsley. Eat right away or refrigerate.

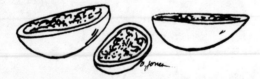

Omelette aux Fines Herbes
(Fresh Parsley, Chervil, and Chives Omelet)

Preparation time: about 4 minutes
Portions: 2
Calories per portion: 100

2 large eggs
¼ teaspoon kosher salt
2 grinds of black pepper

½ tablespoon of combined
    fresh Italian parsley leaves,
    chervil leaves, and chives*
1 teaspoon unsalted butter

Heat a nonstick 6-inch omelet pan or a heavy aluminum or cast iron 6-inch skillet with sloping sides over low heat for 2 minutes.

Beat the eggs in a bowl and season with salt and pepper. Chop the herbs and set aside.

When the omelet pan is hot, put the butter into the pan and turn the heat up to high. Swirl the butter around to cover the entire pan. When the foam subsides, add the eggs and swirl the top of the eggs with a fork, being careful not to scrape the bottom of the eggs. When the eggs start to set around the edges, carefully lift one side with a fork or spatula and let the liquid eggs run underneath. Repeat once or twice until the eggs are completely set with a glossy sheen of uncooked egg on top. Sprinkle the herbs over ½ the omelet. Lift the omelet pan from the stove and hold the serving plate up to meet it. Slide the ½ of the omelet with the herbs onto a plate, then flip the second half over the first to form a half-moon. Serve right away or cool and eat as a cold snack.

Sprout Omelet

Preparation time: about 4 minutes
Portions: 2
Calories per portion: 106

2 large eggs
¼ teaspoon kosher salt
2 grinds of black pepper

1 teaspoon unsalted butter
1 ounce Fresh Bean Sprouts
    (see Index)

Note: Fresh herbs are indispensable in this recipe. If all three are not available fresh, substitute a single fresh herb to make a Tarragon Omelet, a Cilantro Omelet, etc.

Heat a 6-inch nonstick omelet pan or heavy aluminum or cast iron round-sided skillet over low heat for 2 minutes.

Beat the eggs in a bowl and season with salt and pepper.

When the omelet pan is hot, place the butter in the pan and turn the heat up to high. At this point, follow the basic instructions for making an omelet given in the preceding recipe, substituting bean sprouts for the herbs. Turn out onto a plate and eat right away or cool and eat as a cold snack.

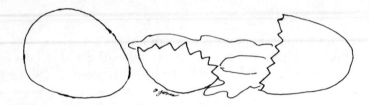

Tomato and Fresh Basil Omelet

Preparation time: about 4 minutes
Portions: 2
Calories per portion: 109

2 large eggs	**3 ounces very ripe tomatoes**
¼ teaspoon kosher salt	**1 teaspoon fresh basil leaves**
2 grinds of black pepper	**1 teaspoon unsalted butter**

Heat a 6-inch nonstick omelet pan or heavy aluminum or cast iron skillet with rounded sides over low heat for 2 minutes.

Beat the eggs in a bowl and season with salt and pepper. Core and halve the tomato. Gently squeeze out the seeds, then chop the tomato into small pieces. Roll the basil leaves into a tight tube and slice thinly. Set aside.

When the omelet pan is hot, place the butter in the pan and turn the heat up to high. At this point follow the basic instructions for making an omelet given in Omelette aux Fines Herbes, substituting the tomato and basil for the herbs. Turn onto a plate and eat right away or refrigerate and eat as a cold snack.

Frittata con Piselli
(Flat Italian Omelet with Peas)

Preparation time: about 15 minutes
Portions: 4
Calories per portion: 82

2 ounces shelled fresh peas or
   2 ounces frozen small peas
¼ ounce yellow onion
½ teaspoon Italian parsley
   leaves

1 tablespoon grated imported
   Parmesan cheese, very
   loosely packed
2 large eggs
¼ teaspoon kosher salt
2 grinds of black pepper
1 teaspoon unsalted butter

Place 1 inch of water in a small saucepan. Cover and bring to a boil. Place the shelled peas in the water and cook, covered, for about 10 minutes, until the peas are tender. If using frozen peas, cook for 3–4 minutes. Drain and save the water for soup.

Chop the onion very fine. Set aside. Chop the parsley and grate the cheese and set aside.

Heat a 6-inch nonstick omelet pan or heavy aluminum or cast iron skillet with sloping sides over low heat for 2 minutes.

Beat the eggs in a bowl and season with salt and pepper. Add the cheese, parsley, onions, and drained peas. Mix gently.

When the omelet pan is hot, turn the heat up to high and place the butter in the pan. Swirl to coat the bottom of the pan. As soon as the butter is melted, pour the egg mixture into the pan. As the sides of the frittata start to set, lift the side up with a fork or spatula so the liquid egg mixture can run underneath. When the bottom has set and is golden brown (the top will still be runny), place a large plate over the pan. With mitts on both hands, lift the pan and flip it upside down so that the frittata is on the plate. Put the pan back on the stove and slide the frittata, uncooked portion on the bottom, back into the pan. When the bottom is golden brown, slide the frittata onto a warm platter and cut it into 4 equal portions or cool and refrigerate and eat as a cold snack.

Peppy Poached Egg

Preparation time: about 5 minutes
Portions: 1
Calories per portion: 130

1 teaspoon white wine vinegar
1 large egg
½ slice Ann's Whole Wheat
    Bread (see Index)

½ teaspoon grated imported
    Parmesan cheese, very
    loosely packed
Dash of paprika

Place a small saucepan of water, covered, over high heat. When the water boils, add the vinegar to the water. Break the egg into a small cup. Remove the cover from the water and stir the water rapidly in a circle with a large spoon to form a vortex. Gently drop the egg into the middle of the vortex. Reduce the heat so that the water is barely simmering. Poach the egg for about 4 minutes, until set and all the white has turned opaque.

While the egg is poaching, toast the whole wheat bread and grate the cheese. When the egg is poached, remove with a slotted spoon and blot the bottom of the spoon on a double thickness of paper towels. Place the egg gently on the bread. Sprinkle with the cheese and a dash of paprika. Eat right away.

Pennsylvania Dutch Pickled Eggs

Preparation time: about 10 minutes
Marinating time: at least 24 hours
Portions: 2
Calories per portion: 85

2 large eggs
Juice from Pickled Beets (see
    Index) or 1 cup canned
    beet juice

GARNISH

**Salt and freshly ground pepper
   or 1 tablespoon Slim
   Snacks Yogurt (see Index)**

If you're using canned beet juice, simmer it with 1 teaspoon of balsamic vinegar, half a bay leaf, 1 clove, and 1 black peppercorn. Simmer the ingredients for 5 minutes, then cool.

Put a small pan of water, covered, on the stove to heat. When it comes to a boil, gently drop the eggs into the water. Reduce the heat and cook at a gentle simmer for 10 minutes. Remove the eggs from the pan and place in a bowl of cold water. After 10 minutes shell the eggs and place in the beet juice. Cover and refrigerate for at least 24 hours before eating. Remove from the juice and slice the egg thin. Garnish with salt and freshly ground black pepper. Or garnish each portion with 1 tablespoon Slim Snacks Yogurt (see recipe), which will add 5 calories to each portion.

FISH AND SEAFOOD SNACKS

Ceviche

This refreshing Mexican appetizer makes a fantastic first course for a fish dinner.

Preparation time: about 15 minutes
Portions: 4
Calories per portion: 74

4 ounces raw sea scallops
**4 ounces cooked medium-
   sized shrimp**
8 ounces ripe tomatoes
**3½ ounces green pepper,
   trimmed of stem, ribs, and
   seeds**

**1½ ounces scallions, green and
   white portion, root end
   trimmed**
**¼ cup fresh lime juice (from
   about 2 limes)**
Kosher salt
Freshly ground black pepper

GARNISH

**1 tablespoon cilantro leaves or
1 tablespoon Italian parsley
leaves chopped with the
zest of ½ lime**

Cut the scallops and shrimp into equal, bite-sized pieces. Cut the tomatoes in half and remove the seeds. Cut into chunks the size of the seafood pieces. Cut the pepper into chunks. Slice the scallion into small circles. Combine all the ingredients except the cilantro in a glass bowl. Season with salt and pepper to taste. Cover and refrigerate for two hours before eating, stirring the mixture every ½ hour.

Just before serving, garnish each portion with freshly chopped cilantro.

Shrimp in Snow Pea Cradles

These shrimp snacks will grace the appetizer tray at your most elegant dinner party.

Preparation time: about 15 minutes
Portions: 20
Calories per portion: 10

**4 ounces fresh snow peas
(Chinese pea pods)
10 cooked medium-sized
shrimp, weighing 4 ounces
½ ounce scallion, white and
green part, trimmed of
root end**

**⅓ cup Slim Snacks Yogurt (see
Index)
2 dashes of Tabasco sauce
Dash of kosher salt**

Break off the ends and remove the strings from the snow peas. Drop them into 2 quarts of boiling salted water and cover until the water returns to the boil. Remove the cover and boil for 1 minute. Drain the peas and then refresh them under cold water. Pat them dry with paper towels. With a sharp paring knife, cut through the destringed side of the pod, being careful not to cut through the sides. The opening should just create a pouch to hold the yogurt filling and the shrimp.

Cut each shrimp in half lengthwise and set aside. Chop the scallion very fine and mix with the remaining ingredients. With a small spoon, spread about ½ teaspoon of the yogurt mixture into the bottom of each snow pea. Place half a shrimp inside each snow pea. Cover and refrigerate.

Tiny Tuna Bundles

These tasty bundles serve triple duty—as a snack, a party hors d'oeuvre, or as a light lunch dish served on a bed of lettuce.

Preparation time: about 10 minutes
Portions: 12
Calories per portion: 22

12 5″ × 5″ red or green leaf lettuce leaves, weighing 5 ounces
1 ounce celery
1 ounce yellow onion
¼ ounce green banana pepper or ¼ ounce green bell pepper, trimmed of stem, ribs, and seeds

¼ ounce Neufchâtel cheese at room temperature
1 6½-ounce can water-packed tuna
¼ teaspoon kosher salt

Wash and dry the lettuce leaves. Set aside. Chop the other vegetables very fine and set aside.

In a small bowl, cream the cheese. Open the tuna can but keep the lid on. Using the thumb to hold the lid down and pressing slightly on it, pour some of the tuna water into the bowl with the cheese. Mix. Keep adding drops of water until the cheese is the consistency of heavy cream. Drain the remaining water into the sink by pressing tightly on the can lid.

Toss the chopped vegetables and the tuna with the dressing. Season with salt. Place 1 tablespoon of tuna salad in the center of each leaf. Fold the right and left sides of the lettuce leaf toward the center until they meet, then fold the bottom and top flap toward the center to form a tight bundle. Place flap side down on a dish and repeat until all the leaves are stuffed. The bundles can be eaten right away or covered and refrigerated for several days.

Trout Steamed in Wine, Fennel, and Shallots

If serving this fish snack for a dinner entree, double the serving portion.

Preparation time: about 10 minutes
Baking time: 3 minutes
Portions: 1
Calories per portion: 109

2 ounces trout fillet (about 3 inches square and 3/8 inch thick)	Kosher salt
	Freshly ground white pepper
	1 teaspoon shallots
2 teaspoons dry white wine	1 teaspoon fresh fennel leaves

Set a heavy baking sheet or a baking stone in the center of the oven and preheat the oven to 500° F.

Fold a 20″ × 12″ piece of foil in half to make a piece 10″ × 12″. Push the sides of the foil up slightly and put 1 teaspoon of the wine in the center. Place the fillet over the wine, then sprinkle lightly with salt and pepper. Chop the shallots and fennel and scatter over the top and pour the other teaspoon of wine over the top. Fold the foil into a tight bundle, taking care to seal the ends well. At this point the fish can either be refrigerated for several hours or baked right away.

Place the fish packet on the baking sheet or stone. Bake for 2 minutes. Flip the packet over and bake for 1 minute. Remove from the oven and eat right away or eat as a cold snack.

Fresh Oysters on the Half Shell

Preparation time: about 5 minutes
Portions: 1
Calories per portion: 44

6 oysters (1 pound 6 ounces   **Lemon wedge**
   with shells)   **Freshly ground black pepper**

Line a fine sieve with cheesecloth and place over a bowl. Holding the oyster in one hand with the more rounded of the two shells on the bottom, use an oyster knife, a v-shaped bottle opener, or a screwdriver to wedge through the shell at the hinge (the more narrow, pointed end of the oyster). Once the hinge is wedged open, use the blade of the oyster knife or another small sharp knife to run across the inside of the flat upper shell. This will cut the muscle holding the oyster to the shell. The muscle will be toward the rounded side opposite the hinge. Once the flat upper shell is loosened, discard it. Set the rounded bottom shell holding the oyster on an oyster plate or a plate of shaved ice. Continue until all the oysters are open. Pour any oyster liquor that has spilled from the oysters over the oysters on the dish. Squeeze lemon over oysters and sprinkle with freshly ground black pepper. Eat right away.

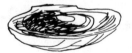

Poached Halibut

Preparation time: about 10 minutes
Portions: 2
Calories per portion: 63

4 ounces fresh halibut or   **½ teaspoon cilantro or Italian**
   turbot fillet, skin attached   **parsley**
1½–2 cups Fish Stock (see   **Lemon or lime wedge**
   Index)

Choose a small skillet or sauté pan just large enough to hold the fish fillet. Estimate how much fish stock is necessary to cover the fillet and heat the stock in the pan. When it reaches a boil, reduce the heat and place the fillet in the stock. Poach in the barely simmering stock for 7–8 minutes. Remove the fillet to a clean cloth and place the fillet skin side up. With a knife or spatula, gently scrape the skin away from the flesh and discard the skin. Using a corner of the cloth as a lifter, flip the fillet onto a spatula, then place on a plate. Garnish with the chopped cilantro and lemon or lime wedge. Eat right away or refrigerate and save for a cold snack.

Cool the stock and strain through a cheesecloth-lined sieve. Refrigerate for several days or freeze.

Marinated Scallop and Vegetable Skewers

This is a great, out-of-the-ordinary dish for a summer picnic or barbecue.

Preparation time: about 5 minutes
Marinating time: 2 hours
Cooking time: about 12 minutes
Portions: 6
Calories per portion: 24

4 ounces bay or sea scallops
2 ounces green pepper,
    trimmed of stem, ribs, and
    seeds

4 ounces small cherry tomatoes
    (about ½ ounce each)

MARINADE

¼ ounce fresh fennel stalk and
    leaves
¾ tablespoon lime juice

½ tablespoon virgin olive oil
Dash of kosher salt
Freshly ground black pepper

If using large sea scallops, cut them in half. Cut the pepper into 1-inch cubes. If the tomatoes are closer to 1 ounce each than they are to ½ ounce, cut them in half.

On a bamboo or nonaluminum metal skewer, thread a piece of pepper, then two pieces of scallop, then a tomato. Repeat twice more on the first skewer, then thread the other 5 skewers in the same way. Place the skewers in a shallow rectangular dish in which they fit tightly. Chop the fennel stalks and leaves. Sprinkle over the top of the scallop skewers. Mix the lime juice and the olive oil. Pour evenly over the scallop skewers. Cover and marinate at room temperature for 2 hours, rotating the skewers several times to coat them with the marinade.

To broil: Position the broiler rack 4 inches from the heat source. Place the skewers on the broiler rack and broil for 8 minutes. Turn the skewers over and broil for 3–4 minutes more. Remove and eat while hot or cool and refrigerate to eat as a cold snack. Allow to come to room temperature before eating.

Chilled Poached Salmon with Dill Sauce

Preparation time: about 10 minutes
Portions: 4
Calories per portion: 106

6 ounces fresh salmon fillet, skin attached	**2½–3 cups Fish Stock (see Index)**

DILL SAUCE

1 tablespoon fresh dill leaves	**Pinch of kosher salt**
6 tablespoons Slim Snacks Yogurt (see Index)	**Freshly ground white pepper**

Choose a small skillet or sauté pan just large enough to hold the salmon fillet. Estimate how much stock is necessary to cover the fillet and heat the stock in the pan. When it reaches a boil, reduce the heat and place the fillet in the stock. Poach in the barely simmering stock for 7–8 minutes. (If the fillet is thicker than 1 inch, increase the cooking time by 2 minutes.) Remove to a clean cloth and place the fillet skin side up. With a knife or spatula, gently scrape the skin away from the flesh and discard the skin. Using a corner of the cloth as a lifter, flip the fillet onto a spatula, then onto a plate. Cool the fillet, then chill in the refrigerator. Strain the stock through a cheesecloth-lined sieve. Cool and refrigerate for several days or freeze.

Chop the dill and mix with the yogurt. Season with the salt and freshly ground white pepper. Place it in a small container and refrigerate.

To serve the fish, divide into 2 portions and spoon sauce over each.

The Shrimp Caper

Preparation time: about 5 minutes (longer if using unshelled shrimp)
Portions: 6
Calories per portion: 49

9½ ounces cleaned shrimp or 12 ounces shrimp in shells
1 ounce yellow onion, chopped
1 bay leaf
3 black peppercorns
1 tablespoon white wine vinegar
½ ounce drained capers
¼ cup Slim Snacks Yogurt (see Index)

If using shrimp in the shell, remove the shells and the vein running down the back of each shrimp.

Place about 1 inch of water in a 10-inch sauté pan with the onion, bay leaf, peppercorns, and wine vinegar. Cover and place over high heat.

Chop the capers and mix with the yogurt. Set aside.

When the water boils, place the shrimp in the pan and cover until the water returns to the boil. Remove the lid and toss the shrimp constantly until opaque (2–3 minutes total cooking time). Remove with a slotted spoon to the yogurt bowl. Toss and eat right away or cool and eat as a cold snack.

POULTRY SNACKS

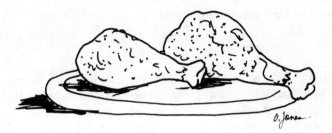

Dijon Chicken Strips

This chicken snack, with a hint of tangy mustard, also makes a fine lunch salad served on a bed of shredded romaine lettuce.

Preparation time: about 15 minutes
Portions: 12
Calories per portion: 16

1½ cups Homemade Chicken
   Stock (see Index)
Salt and freshly ground pepper
5 ounces skinned and boned
   chicken breast

2 tablespoons Slim Snacks
   Yogurt (see Index)
½ teaspoon Dijon mustard
½ teaspoon Italian parsley
   leaves

Heat the chicken stock in a shallow pan just large enough to hold the chicken.

Lightly salt and pepper the chicken breast. When the stock is hot, reduce to a simmer and place the chicken breast in the stock. Poach at a gentle simmer until cooked (about 6 minutes). Remove with tongs and place on paper towels to cool. Strain the stock through a cheesecloth-lined sieve. Cool and refrigerate or freeze.

When the chicken is cool, cut lengthwise into 12 equal strips.

In a shallow bowl, mix the yogurt with the mustard. Lay the chicken strips on top of this mixture and with your hands or 2 forks gently mix the dressing over the strips. Chop the parsley and garnish the chicken with it.

Oriental Chicken Salad

Preparation time: about 5 minutes
Portions: 5
Calories per portion: 82

8 ounces skinned cooked chicken, half white and half dark meat (use chicken from Homemade Chicken Stock or from a roast or broiled chicken that has been seasoned only with salt and pepper)

1½ ounces scallions, white and green part, trimmed of root end
2 ounces Chinese pea pods

DRESSING

1 teaspoon Chinese sesame oil
1 teaspoon vegetable oil
1 teaspoon soy sauce

1 tablespoon white wine vinegar

GARNISH

1 ounce Fresh Bean Sprouts (see Index)

Bring a small pan of water, covered, to a boil.

Cut the chicken into small cubes, cutting the meat across the grain. Wash the scallion and cut into thin slices. Wash the pea pods and remove the tufted end and the string that runs along the straight side of the pod. When the water boils, put in the pea pods and cover. Cook for 1 minute. Drain and rinse in cold water. Lay on a paper towel to dry. Slice each pod on the diagonal into 4 pieces.

In a mixing bowl combine the oils, soy sauce, and wine vinegar with a flat spoon-whisk. Add the remaining ingredients except the bean sprouts. Toss gently to coat the mixture evenly with the dressing. Garnish with the bean sprouts. Serve right away or refrigerate.

Creamy Curry Chicken Salad

Preparation time: about 5 minutes
Portions: 5
Calories per portion: 92

**8 ounces skinned cooked
  chicken, half white and
  half dark meat (use
  chicken from Homemade
  Chicken Stock or from a
  roast or broiled chicken
  that has been seasoned
  only with salt and pepper)**

**1½ ounces scallions, white and
  green part, trimmed of
  root end**
1 ounce celery

DRESSING

**2 ounces Neufchâtel cheese at
  room temperature**

2 tablespoons skim milk
⅛ teaspoon curry powder

Cut the chicken into small cubes, cutting across the grain of the meat. Wash the scallion and cut into thin slices. Wash the celery and chop into small pieces.

In a mixing bowl, cream the cheese. Gradually add the skim milk until the mixture is smooth and liquid. Add the curry powder and mix. Add other ingredients to the dressing and mix to combine. Serve right away or refrigerate.

Chicken Spinach Spirals

This eye-catching rolled chicken breast is as versatile as it is tasty. It can star as the main course for a dinner party (serve a whole roll as a portion) or as a super hors d'oeuvre (just follow the recipe for the snack portion).

Preparation time: about 5 minutes
Baking time: 20 minutes
Portions: 16 spirals
Calories per portion: 20

3 ounces raw spinach leaves, trimmed of stems and spines
2 chicken suprêmes (skinless, boneless breast halves), weighing 4 ounces each
1 small clove garlic
¼ teaspoon kosher salt
2 grinds of black pepper
1 tablespoon grated imported Parmesan cheese, very loosely packed
1 tablespoon dry white wine

Wash the spinach and, with the water clinging to the leaves, place in a small nonaluminum saucepan. Cover and place over high heat. Cook, tossing frequently, until the spinach is wilted. Drain and squeeze dry. Chop very fine and set aside.

Find the fillet strip that runs beside the chicken breast and open out flat. Flatten the chicken suprêmes with a scallopine pounder or a heavy pan. Flatten to a uniform thickness of about ½ inch.

In a small bowl with a heavy spoon or with a mortar and pestle, crush the garlic clove with the salt. Mix until a paste is formed. Add the pepper. Spread the paste evenly over both suprêmes. Place the spinach over each suprême and press to the edge of the top and bottom (the somewhat pointed side and the side that is opposite it). Spread the spinach to within ½ inch of the fillet side and the side that is opposite it.

Sprinkle the Parmesan over the spinach. Beginning with the fillet side, roll each suprême into a tight cylinder. Tuck the little pointed end back toward the center of the cylinder to form a neat package. Tie the bundle with kitchen string at 1-inch intervals. Repeat with the other suprême.

Preheat the oven to 500° F. and place a heavy baking sheet or baking stone in the center of the oven. Place the 2 chicken rolls in the center of a 12″ × 12″ piece of heavy-duty foil. Place the wine around the chicken. Fold the foil to enclose the chicken tightly. Put the bundle on the baking sheet or stone and bake for 20 minutes. Remove and check for doneness by pressing the center of the rolls. If firm to the touch, the rolls are cooked. If not, reseal the foil and bake for 2–3 minutes more.

Remove the chicken from the oven. Unwrap the foil and cut the string around the bundles. Slice each roll into 8 pieces. The spirals can be eaten hot or at room temperature. If refrigerated, allow to come to room temperature before eating.

Roast Chicken Breast with Rosemary and Lemon

Preparation time: about 2 minutes
Roasting time: 45 minutes
Portions: 8
Calories per portion: 22

1 whole chicken breast attached to rib cage, weighing 11½ ounces	**1 teaspoon fresh or frozen rosemary leaves or ½ teaspoon dried**
½ lemon	**Kosher salt**
	Freshly ground black pepper

With a finger, gently loosen the skin covering the breast. Be careful not to loosen the skin at the crest of the breast where the skin is attached to the cartilage. This will anchor the seasonings during the roasting.

Remove the peel and inner white skin from the lemon. Cut into four slices. Tuck two slices under the skin on each half of the breast. Spread the rosemary evenly over the lemon slices. Gently pull the skin down to cover the lemon and rosemary. Sprinkle the underside and topside of the breast lightly with kosher salt and freshly ground black pepper. Place skin side up on a small baking pan. At this point the chicken can be refrigerated or baked right away.

Preheat the oven to 350° F. Place the chicken in the pan in the oven and roast for 45 minutes. Remove from the oven and let rest for 5 minutes. Remove the skin, rosemary, and lemon and discard. Starting at the crest of the breastbone, use a sharp knife and cut down along the rib cage to remove half the breast meat. Repeat with the other half. Cut each half into 4 equal strips. Eat warm or refrigerate for snacking.

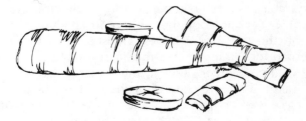

BEEF SNACKS

Beef-Stuffed Cabbage Bundles

Preparation time: about 30 minutes
Cooking time: 1½ hours
Portions: 20
Calories per portion: 69

3 ounces raw rice, enriched or parboiled
4 ounces yellow onion
3 tablespoons Italian parsley leaves

1 pound lean ground beef (85% lean)
1 2¾-pound head of cabbage
1 teaspoon kosher salt
¼ teaspoon freshly ground black pepper

SAUCE

1 large clove garlic
1 28-ounce can tomato puree
¼ teaspoon kosher salt

⅛ teaspoon freshly ground black pepper
½ cup water

Put the rice into a small saucepan and cover with 1½ cups water. Cover, place over high heat, and bring to a boil. Reduce the heat and simmer for 10 minutes, until all the water is absorbed.

Fill a 6-quart pot three-quarters full of water. Cover and set on high heat. Chop the onion and parsley very fine. Combine in a bowl with the ground beef.

Wash the cabbage and remove the stained outer leaves. With a small sharp knife, remove as much of the core as possible. When the pot of water boils, remove the lid and gently drop the cabbage into the pot. Cover and cook the cabbage for 2 minutes. Lift the lid and peel off the top 2 or 3 leaves. Transfer them to a colander. Cover the pan for 2 minutes. Lift the lid and remove 2 or 3 leaves and place in the colander. Repeat until 23 large leaves have been removed. Take out the remainder of the cabbage head and chop coarsely. Place the chopped cabbage in the bottom of a heavy nonaluminum 5- to 6-quart Dutch oven. Set aside.

Chop the garlic very fine. Combine with the tomato puree and season with ¼ teaspoon of salt and ⅛ teaspoon of pepper. Place ½ cup of the puree in the bottom of the Dutch oven with the cabbage. Stir in ½ cup water. Set aside.

Combine the cooked rice, 1 teaspoon salt, and ¼ teaspoon pepper with the meat mixture in the mixing bowl. Mix with the hands until evenly incorporated.

Trim twenty cabbage leaves of about 1 inch of center stem at the base of the leaf. Place 1½ ounces of the meat mixture in the center of each leaf. Fold the bottom section of the cabbage leaf over the stuffing, then fold the sides toward the center. Roll the bundle over the remaining top of the leaf and place fold side down in the pan with the chopped cabbage. Repeat until all the leaves are stuffed. Cover with the remainder of the tomato sauce and the three remaining cabbage leaves. Place a small heat-proof plate over the top and cover with the pan lid. Place over high heat. As soon as the mixture starts to simmer, reduce the heat to medium-low. Cook at a gentle simmer for 1½ hours. The cabbage rolls can be eaten right away or reheated.

Roast Beef Pocket Sandwich with Creamy Horseradish Dressing

Preparation time: about 5 minutes
Portions: 1
Calories per portion: 141

½ of a Whole Wheat Pita, cut to make a semicircle with a pocket (see Index)

1 ounce very lean roast beef, sliced thin
¾ ounce leaf lettuce

DRESSING

2 tablespoons Slim Snacks Yogurt (see Index)

¼ teaspoon prepared horseradish

If desired, wrap the pita in foil and heat for 5 minutes in a 350° F. oven.

Cut the beef into thin strips. Roll the lettuce leaf into a tight tube and slice into thin circles with a sharp knife. Unravel the lettuce into strips.

Mix the yogurt and horseradish. Place the lettuce strips and the beef strips into the pocket in alternating layers. Pour the dressing into the pocket to coat the beef and lettuce. Eat right away. (If preparing the sandwich ahead of time, stuff the pita with the beef and lettuce. Wrap well. Prepare the dressing and package separately. Just before eating, pour the dressing on the sandwich.)

Pita Stuffed with Sesame Beef

Preparation time: about 5 minutes
Portions: 1
Calories per portion: 118

½ of a Whole Wheat Pita, cut to make a semicircle with a pocket (see Index)
¼ teaspoon sesame seeds
¾ ounce leaf lettuce
1 ounce very lean ground beef (85% lean)

¼ ounce yellow onion
Kosher salt
Freshly ground black pepper
Dash of freshly ground cinnamon
1 tablespoon Slim Snacks Yogurt (see Index)

If desired, wrap the pita in foil and heat for 5 minutes in a 350° F. oven.

In a small skillet, toast the sesame seeds until golden brown. Remove from heat and set aside.

Roll the lettuce leaf into a tight tube and slice into thin circles with a sharp knife. Unravel the lettuce into shreds.

Put the beef into a small cold skillet. Place over medium heat. Chop the onion very fine and add to the skillet. Cook, stirring constantly, until the beef is no longer pink. Season lightly with salt and pepper and a dash of cinnamon.

Lay the meat on the bottom of the pita pocket. Lay the lettuce on top of the meat and pour the yogurt over the top. Sprinkle the sesame seeds over the top of the yogurt. Eat right away.

Soft-Shelled Tacos

Most Americans are accustomed to tacos served in a crisp, fried shell, but that is only one way of preparing this popular Mexican snack food. Mexicans also enjoy wrapping piping hot, unfried tortillas around savory fillings to make soft tacos. Diet snackers will love the traditional taco flavor and the untraditional lower calorie count.

Preparation time: about 25 minutes
Portions: 12
Calories per portion: 77

12 Corn Tortillas (see Index)

TACO FILLING

2 ounces yellow onion
1 large clove garlic
12 ounces very lean ground beef (85% lean)
½ teaspoon fresh rosemary or ¼ teaspoon dried

1 teaspoon fresh oregano or ½ teaspoon dried
¼ teaspoon paprika
¼ teaspoon red pepper
¼ teaspoon cumin seeds

GARNISHES

4 ounces leaf or romaine lettuce
4 ounces cheddar cheese

4 ounces tomato
¾ cup Slim Snacks Yogurt (see Index)

Rub the surface of each tortilla lightly with water. Wrap the tortillas in foil and place in a 325° F. oven.

Chop the onion and garlic fine. Press with the beef into a cold heavy 10-inch skillet. Cook over medium-high heat until the bottom is brown (about 10 minutes). Flip the meat and break it up with a spoon. Cook until the meat is no longer red (about 5–8 minutes). Drain the meat through a sieve to remove excess fat. Return the meat to the skillet.

If using fresh herbs, chop fine. Grind the seeds with a mortar and pestle and mix with the herbs. If using dried herbs, grind with a mortar and pestle. Mix with the ground seeds and spices and sprinkle over the beef. Stir the beef and spices and cover the pan. Cook over low heat for 5 minutes.

Roll the lettuce leaves into a tight tube and slice. Separate into shreds. Grate the cheese on the coarse side of a vegetable grater. Core the tomato and cut in half. Squeeze out the seeds. Chop into small pieces.

Remove the tortillas from the oven. Spread out on a flat surface. Divide the beef equally among the tortillas. Garnish with the remaining ingredients and pour 1 tablespoon of yogurt over each taco. Roll one side, then the other, over the center and eat right away.

If you wish to make just 1 taco snack, make it with 1 tortilla and divide the remaining ingredients by 12.

LEGUME SNACKS

Tuscan Bean and Tuna Salad

The cooks in the Italian city of Florence, in the region of Tuscany, make many delicious dishes using dried cannellini beans. This recipe is an adaptation of one of my favorites.

Preparation time: about 10 minutes (with beans already soaked)
Cooking time: about 1½ hours
Cooling time: 30 minutes
Portions: 8
Calories per portion: 83

6 ounces Great Northern dried beans	1 6½-ounce can water-packed tuna
1 ounce yellow onion	1 tablespoon virgin olive oil
1 ounce carrot	1 tablespoon white wine vinegar
1 ounce celery	Dash of kosher salt
1 bay leaf	Freshly ground black pepper
1½ ounces red onion	

Rinse the dried beans well in cold water. Drain and cover with cold water. Let the beans soak at room temperature for at least 5 hours or overnight. Drain the beans and place in a 2-quart saucepan with the coarsely chopped onion, carrot, and celery. Add the bay leaf to the pan and cover with water. Cover the pan and bring to the boil. Reduce the heat to a simmer and cook, covered, for about 1½ hours, or until the beans are tender. Add small amounts of water, if necessary, to keep the beans moist during cooking. Remove lid toward end of cooking time to cook off most of the liquid. When the beans are cooked, remove the vegetables and bay leaf and discard. Allow the beans to cool. At this point they can be refrigerated or the salad can be made right away.

Chop the red onion very fine. Combine in a bowl with the beans. Drain the tuna and add to the bowl. Dress with the oil, vinegar, salt, and pepper. Toss gently. The salad can be eaten right away or refrigerated for several days.

Mid-Eastern Lentil Salad

Preparation time: about 20 minutes plus cooling time
Portions: 8
Calories per portion: 81

6 ounces red lentils
½ ounce yellow onion

1 bay leaf
2 cups cold water

DRESSING

¼ cup Slim Snacks Yogurt (see Index)
1 tablespoon Balsamic vinegar or good-quality aged red wine vinegar

⅓ ounce fresh or frozen chives
¼ teaspoon kosher salt
Freshly ground black pepper
3 ounces romaine lettuce
1 tablespoon fresh mint leaves

Place the lentils in a small saucepan with the onion, bay leaf, and cold water to cover. Cover the pan and place over high heat. When the water boils, reduce the heat and cook at a gentle simmer until the lentils are tender but still very firm (15–18 minutes). Remove from the heat and drain. Spread the lentils on a platter to cool.

Mix the yogurt and vinegar. Chop the chives and combine with the yogurt mixture. Add about ¼ teaspoon kosher salt and some freshly ground black pepper. When the lentils are cool, toss with the dressing. Refrigerate or eat right away. Serve each portion on a leaf of romaine garnished with freshly chopped mint.

6
Beneficial Bread and Grain Snacks

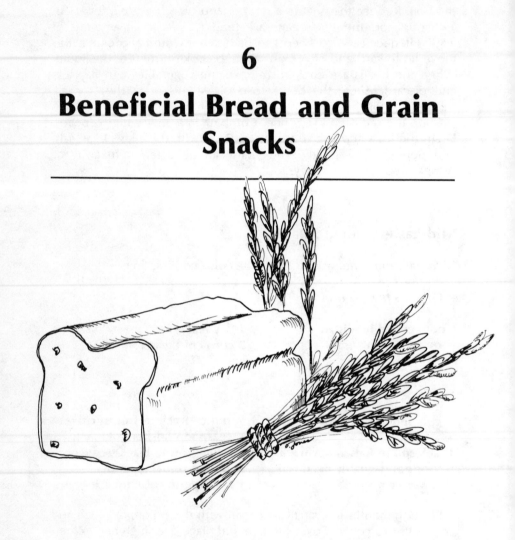

Many dieters deny themselves starchy foods because they mistakenly believe that these foods are more fattening than meats or vegetables. This is just not so. They contain no more calories per ounce than does protein.

Complex carbohydrates, the kind found in whole grains, are vital to good health. Bread and grain snacks impart a psychological feeling of fullness that is important to the dieter. If choosing nutritionally between a snack of a cookie and a slice of whole wheat bread, the whole wheat bread should win hands down. The bread would supply essential nutrients as well as dietary fiber. The cookie would supply lots of refined sugar and fat—in sum, lots of empty calories and very little nutrition.

BAKING BREAD SNACKS—A SATISFYING ADVENTURE

I am always puzzled when I see bread recipes that list sugar as an ingredient. I dislike the cloying flavor that sugar adds to honest wheat bread, and it is not necessary to the rising process as some cooking authorities claim. Bread can be made very successfully (I do it several times each week) using no sugar whatsoever. None of the bread recipes in this chapter contain any sugar. They are also low in fat, which really helps decrease the calorie count.

The most healthful flours are those that are stone-ground from the whole grain. They contain almost all the nutrients of the grain plus the essential dietary fiber. The second best choice is unbleached enriched flour. Some of these recipes use unbleached enriched flour for the sake of variety.

A superior crust and texture for home-baked breads can be obtained with a baking stone, which simulates the results of old-fashioned brick ovens. Baking stones are slabs of clay that have been fired at over 2,000° F. When breads are baked directly on a baking stone or in a pan placed directly on a stone, the bread bakes with a beautiful light texture and crisp crust. The difference in bread baked with a stone is incredible, and it is well worth the effort to find a good stone. They are available in most specialty cookware shops or large department stores. If unavailable in your area, baking stones can be ordered by mail from Old Stone Oven, 616 Davis Terrace, Glen Ellyn, IL 60137.

A large wooden paddle for sliding bread onto the stone is nice but not essential. A piece of cardboard can be used instead.

GRAIN SNACKS: TASTY AND FILLING

Besides the home-baked breads featured in this chapter, I am presenting some tasty grain snacks that deserve more attention from Americans. Cereal grains like bulgur (cracked, parboiled wheat) and kasha (buckwheat groats) not only make fabulous snacks when cooked with stock and aromatic vegetables; they also work into everyday meals beautifully.

Every adult, dieting or not, needs four servings of bread or cereal every day. What better way to get those grains than in mouth-watering home-baked breads and whole-grain cereal snacks?

YEAST BREADS

Ann's Whole Wheat Bread

Preparation time: about 20 minutes
Rising time: about 3½ hours
Baking time: 45–50 minutes
Portions: 40 slices (2 loaves, 20 slices each)
Calories per portion: 87

2 tablespoons unsalted butter
1 cup warm (110° F.) water
1 tablespoon active dry yeast
1 cup warm (110° F.) skim milk
1 teaspoon kosher salt

3 cups whole wheat flour
About 2½ cups all-purpose
    enriched unbleached flour
1 teaspoon vegetable oil

Melt the butter in a small pan and set aside. Heat the water to 110° F. Mix the yeast and ¼ cup of the water with a fork in a small measuring cup. Set aside for about 5 minutes to proof the yeast. (When stirred with a fork it should rise to the surface in spongy blobs.) While the yeast is proofing, heat the milk with the remaining water to 110° F. Mix in the salt.

In a large mixing bowl, combine the yeast water with the milk, water, and salt. Stir. Add the whole wheat flour, 1½ cups at a time, and mix well after each addition. Start adding the all-purpose flour about ½ cup at a time until the mixture is too stiff to mix. Turn out onto a floured surface and begin kneading. Add flour as necessary to keep dough from sticking. Knead the dough until it is smooth and elastic (10–12 minutes). Place the dough in a warm bowl that has been oiled with 1 teaspoon vegetable oil. Run the dough around the bottom of the bowl, then flip over. Cover with plastic wrap and set in a warm, draft-free spot to rise. Let the dough rise until it is doubled in bulk (about 2 hours).

Punch the dough down and turn onto a floured surface. Knead lightly. Divide the dough in ½ with a chef's knife or pastry scraper. Mold into 2 loaves and place in 2 nonstick loaf pans (8½″ × 4½″ × 2½″). Cover and let the loaves rise until doubled in bulk (about 1½ hours).

Twenty minutes before baking, set the rack in the center of the oven. Place the baking stone (if available) on the rack. Preheat the oven to 350° F. Bake the loaves for 45–50 minutes, until they are nicely browned and sound hollow when tapped. Remove from the oven and from the pans. Cool on a wire rack. When cool, the bread can be frozen. Thaw by heating foil-wrapped frozen loaves in a 350° F. oven for 35 minutes or by leaving loaves, unwrapped, at room temperature overnight.

French Bread

Preparation time: about 20 minutes
Rising time: about 2½ hours
Baking time: 45–50 minutes
Portions: 30 slices (2 loaves, 15 slices each)
Calories per portion: 109

1½ tablespoons active dry yeast
2 cups warm (110° F.) water
About 5½ cups all-purpose
    unbleached enriched flour

2 teaspoons kosher salt
1 teaspoon vegetable oil
2 tablespoons cornmeal
Cold water in an atomizer

Sprinkle the yeast over ½ cup of the warm water. Stir gently with a fork and set aside to proof.

In a large mixing bowl combine the yeast water, the remaining 1½ cups warm water, and 2 cups of the flour. Mix well. Add the salt and mix. Continue adding flour, 1 cup at a time, until the dough is too stiff to mix.

Turn the dough onto a floured surface and knead until the dough is smooth and elastic (about 10 minutes). Keep adding flour as necessary if dough sticks to surface. Coat a warm bowl with 1 teaspoon vegetable oil. Run the ball of dough over the bottom of the bowl, then turn over. Cover the dough with plastic wrap and place in a warm, draft-free spot to rise until doubled in bulk (about 1½ hours).

Punch the dough down and knead lightly for 2–3 minutes. Divide the dough into 2 equal portions and shape each into a long thin loaf (about 12 inches long). Scatter the 2 tablespoons of cornmeal evenly down the centers of two baking pans. Place each loaf over the cornmeal. Slash each loaf diagonally at 2-inch intervals. Cover with plastic wrap and set in a draft-free spot to rise until doubled in bulk (35–45 minutes).

Twenty minutes before baking, set the oven rack in the center of the oven. Place a baking stone (if available) on the rack. Preheat the oven to 400° F. Place the baking pans with the loaves on the stone. After 15 minutes open the oven and spray the bread with a fine mist of cold water. Work quickly so as not to lose much heat. Every 15 minutes spray the loaves with cold water (this will make a very crisp crust). Bake the bread for 45–50 minutes, until light brown and hollow-sounding when tapped.

Remove the loaves from the oven and the baking sheets and cool on a wire rack. When the bread is cool it can be frozen. To thaw, bake the foil-wrapped frozen loaves in a 350° F. oven for 35 minutes or leave, unwrapped, at room temperature overnight.

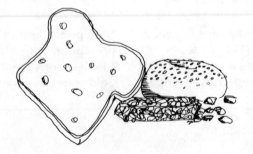

Whole Wheat Pita Bread

These pita breads are as much fun to make as they are to eat. After just a few minutes in a hot oven they magically puff up to form the bread with a pocket.

Preparation time: about 20 minutes
Rising time: about 2½ hours
Baking time: about 3 minutes for each batch; baking will probably have to be done in 2–3 batches
Portions: 24 pita halves
Calories per portion: 73

1 tablespoon active dry yeast
1 cup lukewarm (110° F.) water
1 cup whole wheat flour
1 teaspoon kosher salt

About 2 cups all-purpose unbleached enriched flour
1 teaspoon vegetable oil

Heat the water to 110° F. Dissolve the yeast in ¼ cup of the water and set aside to proof.

Mix the yeast with the remaining water in a large mixing bowl. Mix in the whole wheat flour and the salt. Gradually mix in the white flour, about ¾ cup at a time, until the dough is too stiff to stir and forms a ball. Turn the dough onto a floured surface and knead, adding flour as necessary, until the dough is smooth and elastic (about 10 minutes). Oil a mixing bowl with 1 teaspoon of vegetable oil, then run the dough across the bottom of the bowl and flip over. Cover tightly with plastic wrap and place in a warm, draft-free spot to rise. Let the dough rise until doubled in bulk (about 1½ hours).

When the dough has doubled in bulk, punch it down and turn out onto a lightly floured surface. Knead for 2 minutes. With the palms, roll the dough into a tube shape. With a knife or pastry scraper, cut the dough into 12 equal portions. Form each piece into a ball by pinching the edges together at the bottom. Dust lightly with flour as necessary. Set each ball on a floured surface and press down slightly with the palm to flatten. Cover the balls with plastic wrap that has been lightly dusted with flour. Let them rest for 30 minutes.

After 30 minutes, roll each ball with a rolling pin on a floured surface into a circle about 5–6 inches in diameter. After rolling each ball, place on a floured surface. Cover again with flour-dusted plastic wrap and let rest for 30 minutes.

Twenty minutes before baking the pita bread, place the oven rack in the center of the oven. Place a baking stone or heavy metal baking sheet on the rack. Preheat the oven to 550° F.

After the dough circles have rested for 30 minutes, baking can begin. The pitas will probably have to be baked in several batches, depending on the size of the baking stone or pan used. With a flat wooden paddle or a very large metal spatula dusted with flour, pick up the dough circles 1 at a time and slide onto the baking stone. Place the circles about 2 inches apart. (If using a baking pan, remove from the oven with a pot holder and dust lightly with flour on the spots where the pita rounds will be. Place the rounds on the pan and return to the oven right away.) Once in the oven, the pitas will puff in about 90 seconds on the stone, about 2 minutes on the baking sheet. After another 1½–2 minutes of baking on the stone, the pitas will be done. The baking sheet pitas might require 30 seconds to 1 minute longer. Baking a sample pita is the best way to judge. The pita is done when just the edges of the circle are starting to brown lightly and the pita is still soft to the touch. If overbaked, the pita becomes very brittle. Remove the pitas from the oven and place on a cooling rack. Repeat until all are baked. When they are cool, gently press with the palm to flatten the pitas slightly. Wrap the pitas in foil for 1–2 days or freeze. To thaw, put foil-wrapped frozen pitas in a 350° F. oven for about 20 minutes, until heated through, or leave, unwrapped, at room temperature overnight.

Sourdough Bread

Preparation time: about 30 minutes
Fermentation time: at least 4 days (first batch only)
Rising time: about 2 hours
Baking time: 45–50 minutes
Portions: 32 slices (2 loaves, 16 slices each)
Calories per portion: 123

I. ORIGINAL SOURDOUGH STARTER

½ tablespoon active dry yeast
1 cup warm (110° F.) water

1 cup all-purpose unbleached
enriched flour

With a fork combine the yeast with ½ cup of the warm water. Set aside to proof. Put the flour in a large deep bowl or crock. Add the remaining water to the yeast water and mix with the flour. Cover with a cloth and set in a warm spot to ferment for 2–3 days. (A clear brown liquid will form on the top. Before using the starter, stir the liquid with the rest of the starter.)

II. SECOND FERMENTATION

Original Sourdough Starter
from Step I

1½ cups all-purpose
unbleached enriched flour
1 cup warm (75–85° F.) water

Mix the above ingredients in the crock in which the starter was stored. Cover and place in a warm spot for 24–48 hours.

III. SOURDOUGH BREAD

Starter from Step II, less 1 cup
½ cup warm (75–85° F.) skim
milk
1 tablespoon vegetable oil
½ teaspoon kosher salt

About 4½ cups all-purpose
unbleached enriched flour
2 tablespoons yellow cornmeal
Cold water in an atomizer

Stir the starter in the crock to incorporate any brown liquid that has risen to the top. Remove 1 cup of the starter and place in another crock or jar. Cover and refrigerate. (To keep the starter going, make sourdough bread once a week starting at Step II, using the refrigerated starter as the Original Starter. If you do not make the bread once a week, you can keep the starter going by removing ½ cup of the refrigerated starter and discarding it. Mix ½ cup lukewarm water and ½ cup all-purpose unbleached enriched flour into the starter and rerefrigerate.)

In a large bowl, mix the remaining starter with the warm milk and the oil and salt. Add the flour, 1 cup at a time, until the dough is too stiff to mix. Turn onto a floured surface and knead the dough, working in more flour as necessary, until the dough is smooth and elastic (about 10 minutes).

Divide the dough into 2 portions. Cover and let rest for 15 minutes. With the palms of the hands, roll each portion into a 12-inch loaf. Sprinkle 2 tablespoons of cornmeal down the center of 2 baking sheets. Place 1 loaf on each sheet. Slash the tops of the loaves at 2-inch intervals with a sharp knife. Cover and let rise in a warm spot until doubled in bulk (about 1 hour).

Twenty minutes before baking the bread, position the oven rack in the center of the oven and place a baking stone (if available) on the rack. Set the oven to 375° F.

When the bread has doubled in bulk, place in the oven and bake until well browned and hollow-sounding when tapped (45–50 minutes). After the first 20–25 minutes of baking, spray the loaves at 15-minute intervals with a fine mist of water. This will make a crisp crust.

When the loaves are baked, remove from the oven and place on a cooling rack. Eat right away or freeze. To thaw, place foil-wrapped frozen bread in a 350° F. oven for about 35 minutes or let the bread sit, unwrapped, overnight at room temperature.

Rosemary Pizza Bread

Next is a hearty, flavorful bread—delicious alone or with a hot bowl of soup.

Preparation time: about 20 minutes
Rising time: about 1 hour and 40 minutes
Baking time: 20–25 minutes
Portions: 16
Calories per portion: 77

2 teaspoons active dry yeast
⅔ cup lukewarm (110° F.) water
½ tablespoon fresh or frozen rosemary leaves or ½ teaspoon dried

About 2 cups all-purpose unbleached enriched flour
½ teaspoon kosher salt
2 teaspoons virgin olive oil

Place the yeast in a measuring cup with ½ the water. Stir gently with a fork and set aside until the yeast is proofed. Chop the rosemary leaves very fine and set aside.

When the yeast has proofed, mix the remaining water with the yeast water in a mixing bowl. Add 1 cup of the flour, the salt, and the rosemary. Mix. Keep adding flour and mixing until the dough forms a ball and is too stiff to stir. Turn onto a floured surface and knead, working in flour as necessary to keep the dough from sticking. Knead the dough until it is shiny and elastic (about 10 minutes). Oil a mixing bowl with 1 teaspoon of the olive oil. Run the dough ball around the bowl, then flip over. Cover with plastic wrap and set in a warm, draft-free spot to rise until doubled in bulk (about 1 hour and 15 minutes).

When the dough has doubled, punch it down and turn onto a floured surface. Knead for 2 minutes, then cover with plastic wrap that has been dusted lightly with flour. Let the dough rest for 15 minutes. Meanwhile, place the oven rack in the center of the oven and put a baking stone (if available) or heavy baking pan on the rack. Preheat the oven to 450° F.

Pat the dough into a square with the hands. With a flour-dusted rolling pin, roll the dough into a 12-inch square. Dust a large wooden pizza paddle or piece of sturdy cardboard with flour. Place the dough on the paddle. Brush any flour from the top of the pizza bread and then brush lightly with the other teaspoon of olive oil. Prick the surface of the pizza bread with the tines of a fork at 2-inch intervals. Slide the dough onto the preheated stone or baking sheet. Bake for 20–25 minutes until dough is golden brown. The pizza bread can be eaten warm or cold. To serve, cut into 16 3″ × 3″ squares.

Variations: You can substitute tarragon, basil, oregano, or thyme for the rosemary in this recipe.

Cardamom Oatmeal Bread

Try this delightful, moist bread—it's delicious toasted.

Preparation time: about 20 minutes
Rising time: about 2½ hours
Baking time: 45–50 minutes
Portions: 40 slices (2 loaves, 20 slices each)
Calories per portion: 68

1 cup skim milk
1¼ cups water
1 cup rolled oats (stone-cut is preferable, but the quick-cooking cereal type can be used)

¼ teaspoon fresh cardamom
About 4 cups all-purpose unbleached enriched flour
½ teaspoon kosher salt
1 tablespoon active dry yeast
1 teaspoon vegetable oil

Heat the milk and 1 cup of the water until hot. Mix in a bowl with the oats and set aside to cool to 110° F. Meanwhile, remove the cardamom seeds from the white pods. Discard the pods and grind the seeds in a mortar and pestle. Mix with 1 cup of the flour and the salt. Set aside.

Warm the remaining ¼ cup of water to 110° F. Place the yeast in a measuring cup and pour the water over it. Mix gently with a fork and set aside to proof.

When the yeast is proofed, mix with the oats mixture. Mix in the 1 cup of flour with the cardamom and salt. Continue mixing in flour, 1 cup at a time, until the dough is too stiff to stir. Turn the dough onto a floured surface and knead until the dough is smooth and elastic (about 10 minutes). Sprinkle flour on the surface of the dough as necessary to prevent sticking.

Oil the inside of a mixing bowl with the vegetable oil and run the dough around the inside of the bowl. Flip the dough over and cover the bowl tightly with plastic wrap. Set in a warm, draft-free spot to rise until doubled in bulk (about 1½ hours).

When the dough has doubled, punch it down and turn onto a lightly floured surface. Knead for 2–3 minutes. Divide the dough into 2 portions and shape each portion into a loaf. Place each loaf in a nonstick 8½″ × 4½″ × 2½″ loaf pan. Set in a warm, draft-free spot and cover with plastic wrap. Let rise until doubled in bulk (about 45 minutes to 1 hour).

Twenty minutes before baking, place the rack in the center of the oven. Put a baking stone (if available) on the rack. Preheat the oven to 350° F. Place the loaf pans in the oven and bake for 45–50 minutes, until the loaves are nicely browned and hollow-sounding when tapped. Remove the loaves from the oven and turn onto a cooling rack. When the loaves are cool they can be wrapped tightly in foil and frozen. To thaw, place the foil-wrapped frozen loaves in a 350° F. oven for about 35 minutes or leave, unwrapped, at room temperature overnight.

Fennel Bread

This is one of my favorite breads.

Preparation time: about 20 minutes
Rising time: about 3 hours
Baking time: about 40 minutes
Portions: 40 slices (2 loaves, 20 slices each)
Calories per portion: 59

1 tablespoon active dry yeast
¼ cup lukewarm (110° F.) water
1 cup warm (110° F.) skim milk
2 tablespoons melted unsalted
    butter
½ teaspoon kosher salt

Grated zest of 1 lemon
1 tablespoon lemon juice
1 tablespoon fennel seeds
About 3½ cups all-purpose
    unbleached enriched flour
1 teaspoon vegetable oil

Sprinkle the yeast over the warm water and stir gently with a fork. Set aside to proof the yeast.

In a large mixing bowl, combine the milk, melted butter, salt, lemon juice, lemon zest, and fennel seeds. Stir until well blended. Add the yeast water. Beat in 2 cups of flour. Gradually add enough flour so that the dough forms a ball and is too stiff to mix. Turn onto a lightly floured surface and knead until smooth and elastic (about 10 minutes). Oil a bowl with the vegetable oil and run the dough around the bottom of the bowl. Flip over and cover with plastic wrap. Place the bowl in a warm, draft-free spot to double in bulk (about 2 hours).

When the dough has doubled, punch it down and turn onto a floured surface. Knead lightly. Divide the dough in ½ with a chef's knife or pastry scraper. Mold into loaves and place in 2 nonstick loaf pans (8½" × 4½" × 2½"). Cover and let rise until doubled in bulk (about 1 hour).

Twenty minutes before baking, place the rack in the center of the oven. Put a baking stone (if available) on the rack. Preheat the oven to 350° F.

Bake the loaves on the stone until nicely browned and hollow-sounding when tapped (35–40 minutes). Remove the bread from the oven and from the loaf pans. Cool on a rack. When cool, the bread can be frozen. To thaw, place foil-wrapped frozen loaves in a 350° F. oven for about 35 minutes or leave bread, unwrapped, at room temperature overnight.

Rye Bread with Caraway Seeds

Preparation time: about 20 minutes
Rising time: about 3½ hours
Baking time: 45–50 minutes
Portions: 40 slices (2 loaves, 20 slices each)
Calories per portion: 74

1 tablespoon active dry yeast	1 teaspoon kosher salt
2 cups warm (110° F.) water	3 cups stone-ground rye flour
2 tablespoons melted unsalted butter	About 2½ cups all-purpose unbleached enriched flour
2 teaspoons caraway seeds	1 teaspoon vegetable oil

Mix the yeast in a measuring cup with ½ cup of the warm water. Set aside to proof.

In a large mixing bowl, combine the remaining water, the melted butter, the caraway seeds, and the salt. Mix with the proofed yeast water and the rye flour. Start adding the all-purpose flour, about ¾ cup at a time, until the dough is no longer sticky. Turn onto a floured surface and knead the dough, adding flour as necessary, until smooth and elastic (about 10 minutes). (This dough will not be as elastic as bread made completely from all-purpose flour.) Oil a bowl with the vegetable oil and run the dough around the bowl. Flip over and cover with plastic. Set in a warm, draft-free spot to double in bulk (about 2 hours).

Punch the dough down and turn onto a floured surface. Knead lightly for 2–3 minutes. Divide the dough in ½ and form into loaves. Place each loaf in a nonstick 8½″ × 4½″ × 2½″ bread pan. Cover and let rise until doubled in bulk (about 1½ hours).

Twenty minutes before baking, place the rack in the center of the oven. Put a baking stone (if available) on the rack. Preheat the oven to 350° F.

Bake the loaves until nicely browned and hollow-sounding when tapped (about 45–50 minutes). Remove from the oven and the pans and place on a cooling rack. When cool, the bread can be frozen. To thaw, place the foil-wrapped frozen bread in a 350° F. oven for about 35 minutes or leave the bread, unwrapped, at room temperature overnight.

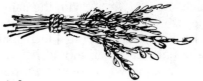

Herb Breadsticks

Preparation time: about 30 minutes
Rising time: about 2½ hours
Baking time: 10–12 minutes
Portions: 52
Calories per portion: 39

1½ cups warm (110° F.) water
1 tablespoon active dry yeast
½ teaspoon kosher salt
3 teaspoons herb seeds
(caraway, fennel, anise, or dill) or 4 teaspoons chopped fresh or frozen herb leaves (basil, oregano, dill, fennel, tarragon, sage, chives, or cilantro)

About 3½ cups all-purpose unbleached enriched flour or substitute whole wheat flour for ½ the flour
1 teaspoon vegetable oil

Heat the water to 110° F. Mix the yeast in ¼ cup of the water and set aside to proof.

When the yeast is proofed, combine with the remaining water, salt, herbs, and 1 cup of flour in a large mixing bowl. Keep adding flour, 1 cup at a time, until the dough is too stiff to mix. Turn the dough onto a floured surface. Knead the dough, adding flour as necessary, until it is smooth and elastic (about 10 minutes).

Oil a mixing bowl with the teaspoon of vegetable oil and run the dough around the bowl. Flip over and cover tightly with plastic wrap. Set in a warm, draft-free spot to rise until doubled in bulk (about 1½ hours).

When the dough has doubled, punch it down and turn onto a lightly floured surface. Knead for 2–3 minutes. Cover the dough with plastic wrap and let it sit for 10 minutes. Divide the dough in half with a pastry scraper or chef's knife. Set one half aside and cover with plastic wrap. Roll the other half into a rectangle 16" × 5". Cut into 13 strips, each about 1½" × 5". With the palms of the hands, roll each strip to a length of about 10 inches. Cut in half and place the strips on nonstick baking sheets about 1 inch apart. Repeat with the other half of the dough. (Each half should yield 26 sticks.) Cover the baking sheets and place in a warm, draft-free spot until doubled in bulk (30–45 minutes).

Twenty minutes before baking, place the rack in the center of the oven. Put a baking stone (if available) on the rack. Preheat the oven to 400° F. Bake the breadsticks until nicely browned (10–12 minutes). Cool on a wire rack. The breadsticks can be frozen when cool. To thaw, place the foil-wrapped breadsticks in a 350° F. oven for about 15 minutes or leave, unwrapped, overnight at room temperature.

QUICK BREADS

Whole Wheat Popovers

Preparation time: about 5 minutes
Baking time: 35 minutes
Portions: 8
Calories per portion: 111

2 teaspoons unsalted butter
2 large eggs
1 cup skim milk

1 cup sifted flour (½ all-
   purpose unbleached
   enriched and ½ whole
   wheat)
⅛ teaspoon kosher salt

Place the baking rack in the center of the oven. Put a baking stone (if available) on the rack. Preheat the oven to 425° F. Two minutes before the popovers are ready to go into the oven, place the popover pan in the oven to heat. (Use a nonstick popover pan, 8 ½-cup muffin tins, or 8 ½-cup custard cups).

Melt the butter in a small pan. Set aside.

In a mixing bowl, beat the eggs. Add the milk and mix. Sift the flour and salt and add to the eggs and milk. Beat well to combine. Mix in the butter. Ladle the batter into the hot popover pan. Bake for 35 minutes.

If the tops of the popovers begin to brown too much, cover lightly with a sheet of aluminum foil. Remove from the oven and from the pans. Cool on a rack. The popovers can be eaten warm or cold.

Irish Soda Bread

Preparation time: about 5 minutes
Bakeng time: 50–55 minutes
Portions: 20 slices
Calories per portion: 92

1½ cups all-purpose
   unbleached enriched flour
1½ cups stone-ground whole
   wheat flour

¼ teaspoon kosher salt
½ teaspoon baking soda
1¼ cups buttermilk

Set the baking rack in the center of the oven and place a baking stone (if available) on the rack. Preheat the oven to 375° F.

In a mixing bowl, combine the dry ingredients. Mix to incorporate. Make a well in the center of the dry ingredients and add the buttermilk. Mix quickly to incorporate the milk evenly. It may be easier to mix with the hands than with a spoon. Form the dough into a loaf shape and place in a nonstick 8½" × 4½" × 2½" loaf pan. Place in the preheated oven and bake for 50–55 minutes, until well browned and a skewer inserted in the center comes out dry. Remove from the oven and the baking pan. Place on a wire rack to cool. The bread can be frozen when cool. To thaw, place the foil-wrapped bread in a 350° F. oven for about 35 minutes or leave, unwrapped, at room temperature overnight.

Corn Tortillas

Preparation time: about 30 minutes
Portions: 12
Calories per portion: 62

1½ cups *masa harina**
¾–1 cup warm water

Mix the *masa harina* and ¾ cup of warm water in a mixing bowl. Gradually add enough extra water to bring the *masa harina* together in a ball. The ball should hold together well but not be excessively wet. (If the tortillas are too wet, they will be impossible to peel from the paper after rolling. If the first batch is too wet, remix the dough, adding a couple more spoons of *masa harina*.)

Turn the dough onto a work surface and shape into a long tube. With a pastry scraper or knife, cut into 12 portions. Roll each portion into a neat ball. As they are formed, lay the balls aside and immediately cover with plastic. When all the balls are formed, press each one in a tortilla press or roll between 2 sheets of waxed paper. (Tortilla presses are available in some specialty cookware shops.) If the edges are ragged, lift the paper and trim the tortilla with a knife.

---

*Note: *Masa harina* (dehydrated masa flour) is made from dried corn that is simmered in lime water until partially soft, then stone-ground and dried. It is available in Mexican groceries and some gourmet food stores.

When all the tortillas are rolled, heat an ungreased griddle or large cast iron skillet over medium heat. When the surface is hot, unpeel as many tortillas as will fit on the griddle without overlapping. Lay them on the griddle. Cook for 1 minute, then flip. Cook 1 minute on the opposite side. Tortillas should puff up slightly. Flip again and cook for another 30–45 seconds. Transfer to a plate or a piece of foil. Stack the cooked tortillas on top of one another. If you are planning to eat these right away or use them in a recipe, keep the stack covered with foil. If planning to refrigerate the cooked tortillas, let them cool by keeping uncovered. Repeat until all the tortillas are cooked. The cooked tortillas can be refrigerated, wrapped tightly, for several days. To reheat, rub the surface of each tortilla lightly with water and wrap in foil. Heat in a 350° F. oven for about 10 minutes.

GRAIN SNACKS

Tabbouleh (Mid-Eastern Bulgur Salad)

Bulgur (or burghul) is cracked wheat that has been hulled and parboiled for quick cooking. Enjoyed widely in Mid-Eastern cooking, the delicious nutlike flavor of bulgur makes an excellent substitute for rice or potatoes. It can be purchased in health food, bulk food, and ethnic food stores.

Preparation time: about 20 minutes
Portions: 6
Calories per portion: 82

3½ ounces bulgur
3 ounces scallions, white and
   green part, trimmed of
   root end

7 ounces tomato
3 tablespoons Italian parsley
   leaves
3 tablespoons fresh mint leaves

DRESSING

1 tablespoon virgin olive oil
2 tablespoons lemon juice

½ teaspoon kosher salt
Freshly ground black pepper

Cover the bulgur with cold water and let sit for 20 minutes. Cut the scallion into thin slices. Core the tomato and cut in half. Gently squeeze out the seeds. Chop the tomato fine. Chop the herbs fine.

Mix the dressing ingredients in a salad bowl with a spoon-whisk.

After 20 minutes, drain the bulgur through a fine sieve. Press to extract all the water. Mix with all the ingredients in the salad bowl. Serve right away or chill before serving. If refrigerated, allow to sit at room temperature for 15 minutes before eating.

Bulgur Pilaf

This is a great side dish for stews and braised meats.

Preparation time: about 20 minutes
Portions: 6
Calories per portion: 113

2 ounces yellow onion
1 small clove garlic
2 teaspoons fresh thyme or ½
   teaspoon dried

5½ ounces bulgur
2 cups hot Homemade Chicken
   Stock (see Index)
½ teaspoon kosher salt

Chop the onion and garlic very fine. If using fresh thyme, chop fine. If using dried thyme, crumble between fingers or with a mortar and pestle. Place all the ingredients in a small saucepan and cover with the hot chicken stock and salt. Stir to combine.

Cover the pan and bring to a boil over medium-high heat. Immediately reduce the heat to low and simmer for 10–12 minutes until the stock is almost absorbed. Remove from the heat and let sit, covered, for 5 minutes before eating.

Mediterranean Pasta Salad

When buying pasta, look for imported brands from Naples or Abruzzo. The texture and flavor are far superior to American-made macaroni pastas.

Preparation time: about 10 minutes
Portions: 10
Calories per portion: 109

½ tablespoon kosher salt
8 ounces imported pasta like
    rotini or penne
1 ounce green or red pepper,
    trimmed of stem, seeds,
    and ribs
1 ounce scallion, white and
    green part, trimmed of
    root end

1 tablespoon fresh or frozen
    oregano or ½ tablespoon
    fresh parsley leaves and 1
    teaspoon dried oregano
    leaves, well crushed with a
    mortar and pestle

DRESSING

3 ounces part-skim ricotta
    cheese
2 teaspoons olive oil
1 tablespoon white wine
    vinegar

2 tablespoons skim milk
¼ teaspoon freshly ground
    black pepper
¼ teaspoon kosher salt

Fill a 6-quart stockpot three-quarters full of water. Cover and set over high heat. When the water comes to the boil, add ½ tablespoon kosher salt to the water. Put the pasta in the pot and stir. Cover the pot until it returns to the boil. Remove the lid and stir again. Reduce the heat slightly and cook until *al dente* (tender but still firm), 7–8 minutes. Drain right away and rinse under cold water. Toss the pasta in the colander to remove as much water as possible. Set aside.

While the pasta is cooking, chop the pepper and scallion into small pieces. Chop the oregano leaves very fine. (If using fresh parsley leaves and dried oregano, chop the parsley and crush the oregano with a mortar and pestle.)

Cream the ricotta in a small bowl. Gradually add the liquid ingredients and mix until the dressing is smooth. Season with salt and pepper.

In a large bowl combine the pasta and the vegetables. Toss with the dressing and the herbs. The salad can be eaten right away or refrigerated. If refrigerated, let the salad sit at room temperature for 15 minutes before eating.

Summertime Tomato Pasta Salad

Preparation time: about 10 minutes
Marinating time: several hours or overnight
Portions: 10
Calories per portion: 102

12 ounces very ripe tomatoes
2 large cloves garlic
1 tablespoon virgin olive oil
1 tablespoon white wine
    vinegar
¼ teaspoon kosher salt
¼ teaspoon freshly ground
    black pepper

2 tablespoons fresh basil leaves
½ tablespoon kosher salt
8 ounces imported penne,
    rotini, or other short pasta

Place a 2-quart pan of covered water over high heat. When the water boils, turn off the heat and place the tomatoes in the pan for 45 seconds. Remove from the pan and place in a bowl of cold water. With a small sharp knife, remove the cores and skins from the tomatoes. Halve them and squeeze gently to remove the seeds. Chop the tomatoes into small pieces and place in a glass bowl.

Smash the garlic cloves with a heavy knife and remove the skins. Slice the garlic into 6 pieces. Add the garlic slices to the tomatoes. Season with the olive oil, vinegar, salt, and pepper. Bunch the basil leaves together and roll into a tight tube. Slice thinly and mix with the tomatoes. Cover the tomatoes and marinate in the refrigerator for several hours or overnight.

To cook the pasta and assemble the salad: Fill a 6-quart stockpot three-quarters full of water. Cover and set over high heat. When the water comes to the boil, add ½ tablespoon of kosher salt. Put the pasta in the water and stir. Cover the pan and return to a boil. Remove the lid and lower the heat slightly. Stir the pasta and cook until it is *al dente* (tender but still firm), 7–8 minutes. Drain in a colander and rinse well with cold water. Toss to remove as much water as possible.

Remove the garlic slices from the tomatoes and discard. Toss the tomato marinade and the pasta together. Eat right away or return to the refrigerator for several days. If refrigerated, allow to sit at room temperature for about 15 minutes before eating.

Pasta Parmesan

Preparation time: about 8 minutes
Portions: 2
Calories per portion: 85

1 teaspoon kosher salt
1½ ounces of imported pasta
such as spaghetti, linguini,
rotini, or penne
¼ cup Homemade Chicken
Stock (see Index)

1 tablespoon grated imported
Parmesan cheese, very
loosely packed
Freshly ground black pepper

Bring a 4-quart pan of covered water to the boil. Add the kosher salt. Put the pasta in the water and stir. Cover the pan. When the water returns to the boil, remove the lid and stir the pasta. Reduce the heat slightly and cook for about 5 minutes.

Drain into a colander and shake to remove excess water. Return the pasta to the cooking pot and add the chicken stock. Toss for 3–4 minutes over medium heat until the stock begins to thicken and coat the pasta. Place the pasta in a bowl and garnish with cheese and freshly ground black pepper.

Kasha in Chicken Stock

Buckwheat groats, or *kasha* as they are often labeled, are a staple of Eastern European and Russian cooking. The groats are the roasted grains of the buckwheat plant and are available whole, medium-ground, and finely ground. They have a rich, hearty taste that makes a fabulous change-of-pace side dish.

Preparation time: about 7 minutes
Portions: 2
Calories per portion: 84

½ cup Homemade Chicken
Stock (see Index)
⅛ ounce yellow onion

1½ ounces buckwheat groats,
coarse or medium
Pinch of kosher salt

GARNISH

**½ teaspoon Italian parsley
   leaves**

   Put the stock in a small saucepan. Cover and set over medium
heat. Chop the onion very fine.
   When the stock boils, put the onion, groats, and salt into the pan
and stir. Cover and return to the boil, then reduce the heat to a
gentle simmer. Cook for 5 minutes or until all the stock is absorbed.
Chop the parsley and sprinkle over the kasha as a garnish.

Armenian Rice Pilaf

   Armenian Rice Pilaf is a wonderful accompaniment to chicken
sautés or lamb braises.

   Preparation time: about 35 minutes
   Portions: 6
   Calories per portion: 90

1 ounce vermicelli
¾ ounce yellow onion
1 teaspoon unsalted butter
**1¼ cups Homemade Chicken
   Stock (see Index)**

**½ cup enriched, parboiled
   long-grain rice**
¼ teaspoon kosher salt
**Pinch of freshly ground white
   pepper**

   Preheat the oven to 350° F. Break the vermicelli into small pieces.
Spread on a baking sheet and place in the oven until golden brown
(about 15 minutes). Remove the vermicelli. (This step can be done
in advance and the toasted vermicelli stored in an airtight container.)
   Chop the onion very fine. In a 2-quart saucepan, melt the butter.
Stew the onion in the butter until soft (about 5 minutes). Heat the
chicken stock in a small pan. Add the vermicelli and rice to the
onion and toss until coated with butter. Add the hot stock, salt, and
pepper. Cover and place over high heat. Bring to a boil and reduce
heat right away. Cook at a gentle simmer for 15 minutes. Remove
from heat and let sit 5 minutes. Serve right away or eat at room
temperature.

7

Sensuous Sweet Snacks

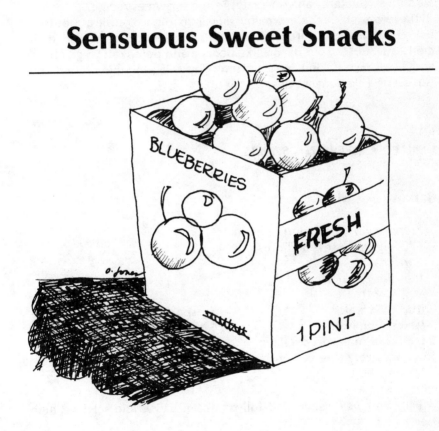

For many dieters, sweets and desserts seem to be the hardest habit to kick. If you are among them, this chapter is for you. These sensuous sweet snacks contain lower doses of sugar and honey than regular desserts and, wherever possible, I have included more nutritious ingredients than are usually found in desserts. For example, I have substituted whole wheat flour and carob (contains less fat and is sweeter than chocolate) in the brownies recipe.

These sweets include creamy puddings, light soufflés, mousses, baked meringues, refreshing sherbets, frozen custards, and delicious quick breads in flavors like banana and pumpkin. So go ahead and enjoy—you don't have to deny yourself everything when you can savor a slim-snacks dessert.

CHILLED AND FROZEN SWEETS

Banana Soufflé

Preparation time: about 5 minutes
Chilling time: several hours
Portions: 8
Calories per portion: 41

¼ cup cold water
1 tablespoon honey
1 teaspoon unflavored gelatin
13 ounces very ripe bananas
1 lemon wedge

1 teaspoon vanilla extract
2 large egg whites at room temperature
Dash of cream of tartar

Fill a small saucepan half full of water. Cover and set over high heat.

In a small measuring cup mix the water and honey. Stir to dissolve the honey. Sprinkle the gelatin over the top of the honey water and place the cup, double boiler style, in the pan of hot water. Remove from the heat and let stand until gelatin dissolves (6–7 minutes).

Puree the bananas in a blender or food processor fitted with the steel blade or through a food mill. Add the lemon juice from the lemon wedge and the vanilla. Mix and set aside.

Whip the egg whites with an electric mixer until they start to foam. Add a dash of cream of tartar and continue beating until they are stiff but not shiny.

Mix the gelatin water with the pureed bananas. Stir ¼ of the whipped egg whites into the banana mixture. Gently place the remaining whites on top of the banana puree and fold the whites into the puree. Chill in a glass dish. To serve, spoon portions from the dish.

If serving this snack for a guest dessert, it will make 4 portions: Fit 4 ¾-cup soufflé molds or custard cups with foil collars about 1 inch above the top of each dish. Tie with kitchen string to secure. Gently spoon the soufflé into each dish. Cover and chill until firm. Serve each soufflé with 4 tablespoons of Delectable Whipped Dairy Topping (see Index). Remove foil collars before serving.

Four dessert portions with topping will have 89 calories per portion.

Raspberries in a Cloud

Preparation time: about 5 minutes
Chilling time: several hours
Portions: 16
Calories per portion: 16

1 teaspoon unflavored gelatin	**Dash of cream of tartar**
¼ cup cold water	**3 tablespoons granulated sugar**
4 large egg whites at room temperature	**8 ounces cleaned raspberries**

Place a small pan of water, covered, over high heat. Sprinkle the gelatin powder over the ¼ cup of water in a small heatproof cup. Place the cup in the hot water, double boiler style. Turn off the heat and allow to sit until the gelatin dissolves (about 5 minutes).

Whip the egg whites with an electric beater until they start to foam. Add the cream of tartar and continue beating. Gradually add the sugar, a little at a time, and beat the egg whites until stiff but not shiny. During the last few minutes of beating, pour the melted gelatin into the egg whites. Gently fold the berries into the meringue. Pour into an 8-inch square glass dish. Cover and chill until set (several hours). Cut into 16 squares to serve.

Divine Blueberry Mousse

Preparation time: about 10 minutes
Chilling time: several hours
Portions: 8
Calories per portion: 46

¼ cup apple juice
1 tablespoon honey
1 teaspoon unflavored gelatin
8 ounces blueberries
1 cup Slim Snacks Yogurt (see Index)

2 large egg whites at room temperature
Dash of cream of tartar

Cover a small pan of water and place over high heat.

Mix the apple juice and the honey in a small cup. Stir to dissolve the honey. Sprinkle the gelatin over the top and place the cup in the small pan of hot water, double boiler style, until the gelatin dissolves (6–7 minutes).

Puree the berries in a blender or food processor fitted with the steel blade or through a food mill. Strain through a fine sieve to remove the skins. Press well with a spatula to remove all the juice. Discard the solids.

Stir the yogurt into the berry juice. When the gelatin is melted, add it to the berry juice and yogurt mixture. Stir to incorporate gelatin.

With an electric mixer, beat the egg whites until they start to foam. Add a dash of cream of tartar and continue beating until the whites are stiff but not dry. Fold into the berry-yogurt mixture. Gently pour or spoon the mousse into a 3-cup bowl. Cover and chill until set (several hours). To serve, spoon the portions from the bowl.

Sunshine Gelatin

Preparation time: about 8 minutes
Chilling time: several hours
Portions: 4
Calories per portion: 93

¼ cup cold water
2 tablespoons honey
1 envelope unflavored gelatin

Zest from 1 orange
1¾ cups freshly squeezed
    orange juice

Put a small pan of water, covered, over high heat. Mix the cold water and the honey in a small cup. Sprinkle the gelatin over the top. Place the cup in the hot water, double boiler style. Turn off the heat and let the gelatin sit until dissolved (6–7 minutes).

Grate the orange zest on the fine side of a grater or with a citrus zester. After removing with a zester, chop the zest very fine.

Squeeze the orange juice, then combine with the chopped zest. Stir in the melted gelatin and honey. Pour into a small bowl or into 4 glass dishes. Cover and chill until set (several hours).

Strawberry Sherbet

A cool, refreshing summer treat, this is the essense of vine-ripened strawberries. The surprising addition of black pepper enhances the sweetness of the berries.

Preparation time: about 5 minutes
Freezing time: about 5 hours
Portions: 8
Calories per portion: 53

1 pint very ripe strawberries
½ cup water
¼ cup honey

2 tablespoons lemon juice
Up to ⅛ teaspoon finely
    ground black pepper

Clean the strawberries and remove the tops. Puree in a food processor fitted with the steel blade, in a blender, or through a food mill or sieve. Heat the water and add the honey, stirring until melted. Mix with the strawberry puree. Add the lemon juice and black pepper to taste. Place the sherbet mixture in a flat glass or ceramic dish (about 10 inches square). Cover and place in the freezer.

After 45 minutes, remove the dish from the freezer and, with a large spoon, scrape the sides and bottom of the dish to mix any partially frozen sherbet with the still-liquid sherbet in the center.

Repeat this every 45 minutes until the sherbet is solid. The sherbet will be the smoothest at this time. If it must wait for 24–48 hours before serving, remove from the freezer and puree the frozen sherbet in a food processor with the steel blade or in the blender until smooth. Serve right away. (The sherbet can also be made in an ice cream or sherbet machine following manufacturer's instructions.)

Lime Ice

Preparation time: about 1 minute
Portions: 1
Calories per portion: 37

4 tablespoons lime juice
½ teaspoon honey
4 ice cubes (1″ × 1″ × ¾″)

Place the lime juice in a food processor or blender. Add the honey and process until frothy (about 30 seconds). With the machine running, add the ice cubes through the feed tube. Process until finely chopped and a slushy consistency. Pour the ice into a small dish or cup and eat right away.
Variations: Substitute 4 tablespoons of lemon or orange juice for the lime juice.

Frozen Orange Custard

Preparation time: about 10 minutes
Freezing time: several hours
Portions: 8
Calories per portion: 76

Juice of ½ lemon plus enough   **Zest of 1 orange**
**   orange juice to make 1 cup**   **1 large egg yolk**
¼ cup honey   **1¼ cups whole milk**

Squeeze the lemon and orange juices and mix with the honey in a heavy nonaluminum saucepan. Grate the orange zest very fine and add to the liquid. Beat the egg yolk into the mixture and cook over medium-low heat until the mixture starts to thicken. (It will register 165° F. on an instant-reading thermometer.) Remove from the heat and stir rapidly to stop cooking. Pour into a bowl and set aside to cool.

When the mixture is cool, stir in the milk, cover, and place in the freezer. After about 45 minutes, remove the custard and scrape the sides and bottom with a large spoon, mashing the frozen portion and mixing it with the liquid portion. Repeat every hour until the mixture is at the soft freeze stage. Place in a blender or the bowl of a food processor and puree until smooth. Return to the freezer for 1 hour. The custard is best if eaten at this stage, before large ice crystals form. If the custard stays in the freezer for several days, remove it and let sit at room temperature for about 30 minutes. Spoon into a food processor fitted with a steel blade. Puree until smooth. Eat right away. (The custard can also be made in an ice cream machine following manufacturer's instructions.)

PUDDINGS AND PUREES

Pumpkin Puree

Preparation time: about 40 minutes
Yield: 4 cups of puree

1 3¾-pound pumpkin

Choose a deep pan with a wide surface area. Fill with several inches of water and then place a steamer rack in the pan. (A wok with a steamer rack is excellent because of the large steaming surface. The pumpkin should be steamed in one layer, so, depending on the size of the pan, it may have to be steamed in 2 batches.)

Cover the pan and place on the stove to heat.

If the pumpkin is dirty, wash it under cold water and dry. With a large sharp knife, cut the pumpkin in half through the stem and scoop out the seeds and stringy center flesh. (Save the seeds to roast according to the technique for Roasted Squash or Pumpkin Seeds—see Index.) Cut each half in half again and, with a small sharp knife, peel away the tough outer skin. Cut the pumpkin flesh into 1-inch cubes. When the water comes to the boil, place a solid layer of pumpkin cubes on the steamer rack and replace the lid. Reduce the heat slightly. Steam the pumpkin until it is tender (15–20 minutes). Check by inserting a small sharp knife into the pumpkin.

When the pumpkin is cooked, remove and place on a kitchen towel or paper towels, then puree the pumpkin in a blender or through the fine disc of a food mill or in a food processor fitted with the steel blade. Puree until smooth, scraping down the sides of the bowl as necessary. At this point the pumpkin can be used in a recipe (the two following recipes, Pumpkin Bread, and Pumpkin Soup) or cooled and refrigerated for several days.

Pumpkin Pleaser

Preparation time: about 2 minutes
Portions: 1
Calories per portion: 49

½ cup Pumpkin Puree (see preceding recipe)

¼ teaspoon coriander seeds
½ teaspoon pure maple syrup

If the puree has been refrigerated, gently reheat it in a small saucepan until warm. Place the coriander seeds in a small heavy skillet and toast over medium heat until lightly browned. Grind the seeds with a mortar and pestle.

Place the puree in a small dessert bowl and mix with the ground seeds. Drizzle maple syrup over the top. Eat right away.

Pumpkin Custard

Preparation time: about 5 minutes
Baking time: about 1 hour
Portions: 6
Calories per portion: 78

½ teaspoon cinnamon
¼ teaspoon gingerroot
Zest of 1 orange
2 large eggs
2 tablespoons pure maple
    syrup

1 cup Pumpkin Puree (see
    Index)
1 cup skim milk
1 teaspoon pure vanilla extract

Select a 4-quart glass or ceramic baking dish and another large dish in which it will fit with about a 2-inch area between the sides of the baking dishes. Bring a kettle of water to the boil. Preheat the oven to 350° F.

Grind the cinnamon. Grate the gingerroot very fine. Grate the orange zest very fine and set aside.

In a mixing bowl, beat the eggs until smooth. Blend in the maple syrup. Mix in the pumpkin puree, the skim milk, and the seasonings. Mix well, then pour into a 4-quart baking dish or 6 ½-cup custard cups. Pour the hot water into the outer baking dish and fill until the water comes three-quarters up the sides of the inner dish. Place the custard in its hot water bath in the oven and bake until a knife inserted in the center comes out clean (about 1 hour for a baking dish, 30–35 minutes for individual custard cups). Remove from the oven. The custard can be served hot, warm, or cold.

Old-Fashioned Rice Pudding

Preparation time: about 30 minutes
Portions: 10
Calories per portion: 59

1 tablespoon honey
3 cups skim milk
¾ cup rice, parboiled or
    enriched

1 ounce dark raisins
½ teaspoon nutmeg

In a 4-quart heavy saucepan, combine the honey and ½ cup of the milk. Stir over medium heat until the honey is dissolved. Add the remaining milk and the rice. Stir to combine. Cover and set over high heat. Watch very carefully for the milk to come to a boil (about 5 minutes). As soon as it does, reduce the heat to medium-low and set the pan lid ajar. Cook, removing the scum from the top of the milk every 5 minutes or so.

While the rice is cooking, chop the raisins into very small pieces. Add to the rice and milk after 20 minutes of cooking time.

Grate the nutmeg on the fine side of a cheese grater or on a special nutmeg grater.

The rice should be done after 25 minutes of cooking time. It should be soft and creamy in consistency. Remove from the heat and stir in the nutmeg. Serve lukewarm or cool and refrigerate. If refrigerated, allow the pudding to sit at room temperature for 15 minutes before eating.

Coffee Custard

Preparation time: about 5 minutes
Chilling time: several hours
Portions: 4
Calories per portion: 59

½ tablespoon unflavored gelatin
3 tablespoons cold water
½ cup skim milk
½ cup strong brewed coffee (French roast or espresso)

2 large egg yolks (refrigerate or freeze the whites for use in meringue recipes)
2 teaspoons honey
1 tablespoon 80-proof rum

Heat a small pan of water. Sprinkle the gelatin over the cold water in a small cup. Set the cup in the pan of hot water, double boiler style, and set aside until the gelatin melts (5–6 minutes).

In a small pan, heat the milk and coffee until hot. In a small nonaluminum saucepan, whisk the egg yolks and honey together. Gradually pour the hot milk and coffee into the pan with the eggs and honey. Whisk to combine. When the mixture is smooth, use a large spoon to constantly stir the custard over medium-low heat. Cook for 3–4 minutes until the custard starts to thicken (165° F. on an instant-reading thermometer). Remove the custard from the heat and whisk in the rum and the dissolved gelatin. Whisk for 1–2 minutes to cool the custard and stop the cooking. Spoon into 4 small custard cups and cool. Cover and chill for several hours in the refrigerator before eating.

Pear Puree with Vanilla Custard Sauce

Preparation time: about 25 minutes
Portions: 6
Calories per portion: 113

VANILLA CUSTARD SAUCE

¾ cup skim milk
3 large egg yolks (refrigerate or
    freeze the whites for use in
    meringue recipes)
1 tablespoon honey
1 teaspoon vanilla

PEAR PUREE

2 pounds pears
¼ teaspoon nutmeg

To prepare the custard sauce: Heat the milk in a small nonaluminum saucepan. In a heavy 2-quart nonaluminum saucepan, whisk the egg yolks and honey until smooth. Whisk in the hot milk until smooth. Place the pan over medium heat and stir constantly with a spoon until the custard starts to thicken (it will register 165° F. on an instant-reading thermometer). Remove from heat immediately and whisk to stop the cooking. Whisk in the vanilla and set the custard sauce aside.

Peel the pears. Cut into quarters and remove the cores. Cut each quarter into 3 chunks. Place the pears in a heavy 2-quart saucepan with about ½ inch of water in the bottom of the pan. Cover and place over high heat. When the water boils, reduce the heat to low and cook off any excess liquid in the pan. Toss the pears so they do not scorch.

Puree the pears in a blender or food processor fitted with the steel blade or through a food mill. Season with freshly grated nutmeg.

Serve in small bowls with the custard sauce poured over the pear puree. This snack can be served warm or cold.

Red Raspberry Fool

This snack is a delightfully light adaptation of an old English fruit puree and egg custard dessert.

Preparation time: about 20 minutes
Chilling time: several hours
Portions: 10
Calories per portion: 96

CUSTARD

1¼ cups skim milk
2 tablespoons honey
2 strips lemon rind
1 strip orange rind

3 large egg yolks (refrigerate or freeze the whites for use in meringue recipes)
2 tablespoons arrowroot powder or cornstarch

Heat all but 1 tablespoon of the milk, the honey, and the citrus rinds in a nonaluminum saucepan over moderately low heat. Stir to dissolve the honey. When the milk is hot, cover the pan, remove from heat, and set aside.

Whisk the egg yolks, the arrowroot powder, and the remaining tablespoon of milk in a bowl until blended. Slowly pour in the hot milk, whisking the mixture as you pour.

Strain the mixture back into the saucepan through a fine sieve and cook it over low heat, stirring constantly. Cook until the custard is thickened (7–10 minutes). Pour into a bowl and cool it. Cover with plastic wrap and chill the custard.

RASPBERRY PUREE

24 ounces red raspberries
3 strips lemon rind

2 tablespoons honey
2 tablespoons orange liqueur

Combine the berries, lemon rind, and honey in a heavy saucepan and cook, covered, over moderately low heat for 5 minutes. Uncover the pan and boil gently until the mixture is thick and sticky (about 15 minutes). Stir the mixture frequently in the early stage of cooking.

Remove the lemon rind and force the berries through the fine disc of a food mill or puree in a blender or food processor, fitted with steel blade. If desired, strain through a fine sieve to remove seeds. The consistency should be that of a thick fruit sauce. If it is not thick enough, boil the puree a little more, stirring often. Don't let the mixture become too thick, because it will thicken considerably when chilled. Remove from the heat and add the orange liqueur. Cool the mixture, then cover and chill for several hours.

To serve the fool: Remove the custard and the raspberry puree from the refrigerator. Beat both with a large spoon to smooth the mixtures. Fold the raspberry puree into the custard. Do not fold completely—the fool should have a streaked appearance with swirls of fruit in the custard. Serve right away or rechill and serve later.

Lime Custard

Preparation time: about 5 minutes
Baking time: about 35 minutes
Portions: 8
Calories per portion: 60

Zest of 1 lime　　　　　　　　**2 cups skim milk**
2 large eggs　　　　　　　　　**1 teaspoon pure vanilla extract**
2 tablespoons honey

Choose a baking pan that will hold 8 ½-cup custard cups with 2 inches of space all around each cup. Bring a kettle of water to the boil and preheat the oven to 350° F.

Grate the lime zest on the fine side of a grater or remove in strips with a citrus zester. Chop the strips fine with a knife.

Beat the eggs in a mixing bowl. Blend in the honey until well incorporated. Mix in the milk, vanilla, and lime zest. Ladle the mixture into the custard cups, filling about three-quarters full. (The lime custard can also be baked in a 4-quart glass or ceramic baking dish.) Fill the outer baking pan with hot water until the water level is three-quarters up the side of the custard cups or baking dish.

Bake until a knife inserted in the center comes out clean (about 35 minutes for individual custard cups and 1 hour for a single baking dish). Remove from the oven. Eat warm or cold.

Variations: Substitute orange, lemon, or a combination of lime, lemon, and orange zest for the lime zest in the recipe.

Orange Dream

This snack is a luscious treat that tastes like orange whipped cream.

Preparation time: about 3 minutes
Portions: 4
Calories per portion: 24

Zest of 1 orange
⅓ cup freshly squeezed orange juice (juice from 1 medium orange)

⅔ cup skim milk
3 ice cubes (1″ × 1″ × ¾″)

Remove the zest from the orange and chop very fine or grate on the fine side of a vegetable grater. Place the orange juice, milk, and grated zest in the work bowl of a food processor fitted with a steel blade. Process to mix. With the machine running, add the ice cubes, 1 at a time, to the milk and juice. Process for about 2 minutes, until the mixture is very thick. Eat right away.

BAKED SWEETS

Meringue Shells

Preparation time: about 5 minutes
Baking time: 1 hour and 45 minutes
Drying time: several hours
Portions: 8
Calories per portion: 5

1½ tablespoons confectioner's sugar

2 large egg whites at room temperature
⅛ teaspoon cream of tartar

Preheat the oven to 190° F.
Pass the confectioner's sugar through a fine sieve. Place the egg whites in a mixing bowl. Beat with an electric mixer until foamy,

then add the cream of tartar. Whip the whites until soft mounds form, then gradually add the confectioner's sugar. Continue beating the whites until stiff but not shiny. Drop 8 large spoonfuls of the meringue onto a nonstick baking sheet or a regular baking sheet lined with parchment paper.

With a teaspoon, gently round off the sides of each mound, then make an egg-shaped depression in the center of each. Bake in the preheated oven for 1 hour and 45 minutes. Turn off the oven and allow the meringue shells to dry in the oven for several hours with the oven door partially open. Gently remove the meringues from the baking sheet with a metal spatula. (If baked on parchment paper, gently remove the meringues with the fingers of 1 hand while peeling the paper away with the other.) Store in an airtight tin or eat right away.

Fresh Fruit in Meringue Shells

Preparation time: about 3 minutes (with meringue shells baked)
Portions: 8

8 ounces fresh sliced fruit that has been trimmed of skins and seeds

8 Meringue Shells (see preceding recipe)
½ recipe Delectable Whipped Dairy Topping (see Index)

Wash and slice the fruit. Small berries can be left whole if desired. Spoon the fruit equally into the meringue shells. Top with equal portions of the Delectable Whipped Dairy Topping.

Fruit Flavor	Calories per portion
Strawberries in Meringue Shells	25
Blueberries in Meringue Shells	32
Raspberries in Meringue Shells	33
Peaches in Meringue Shells	22

Carob-Dusted Meringue Puffs

Preparation time: about 5 minutes
Baking time: 1 hour and 30 minutes
Drying time: several hours
Portions: 16
Calories per portion: 5

**2 large egg whites at room
    temperature**
⅛ teaspoon cream of tartar

2 teaspoons carob powder
**3 tablespoons confectioner's
    sugar**

Preheat the oven to 190° F. Prepare the egg whites exactly as in the Meringue Shells recipe, mixing the carob powder with the confectioner's sugar before adding to the egg whites.

Drop the prepared meringue into 16 small mounds on a nonstick baking sheet or a baking sheet lined with parchment paper. Bake for 1 hour and 30 minutes. Turn off the oven and allow the puffs to cool in the oven with the door partially opened. Remove the puffs gently from the baking sheet and store in an airtight tin or eat right away.

Pineapple Clouds

Preparation time: about 5 minutes
Baking time: 20 minutes
Portions: 4
Calories per portion: 105

**4 pineapple slices, each
    weighing 5½ ounces**
½ ounce walnuts

**2 large egg whites at room
    temperature**
Dash of cream of tartar

Heat the oven to 300° F.

With a large chef's knife, cut the bottom from the pineapple. Leaving the skin on, cut 4 slices, each about 4½ inches wide and ½ inch thick. With a small sharp knife, cut out a slight depression in the hard center core of each slice, but don't cut all the way through. Lay the slices on a baking sheet.

Grind the nuts in the food processor with the steel blade or in a nut grinder. Grind very fine and set aside.

With an electric mixer, whip the egg whites until they start to foam. Add a dash of cream of tartar to the whites and continue beating until they are stiff but not shiny.

Spoon the meringue equally over each pineapple slice and spread to cover the entire slice. Sprinkle each slice with the ground walnuts. Place in the oven and bake until the meringue is golden brown (about 20 minutes). Serve hot or at room temperature.

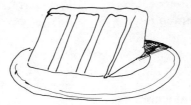

Orange-Rum Banana Bake

Preparation time: about 1 minute
Baking time: 12 minutes
Portions: 2
Calories per portion: 63

1 6-ounce banana	**1 tablespoon 80-proof dark**
2 tablespoons orange juice	**rum**
	Freshly grated nutmeg

Peel banana and slice in half lengthwise. Place in a small baking dish. Mix the orange juice and rum and pour over the banana. Bake in a preheated 400° F. oven for 12 minutes. Remove and dust lightly with freshly grated nutmeg. Serve right away.

CAKES, COOKIES, AND SWEET BREADS

Lemon Spongecake

Preparation time: about 10 minutes
Baking time: about 1 hour
Portions: 14
Calories per portion: 119

2 teaspoons unsalted butter
2 tablespoons cornstarch mixed
   with enough all-purpose
   unbleached enriched flour
   to make 7 ounces
2 tablespoons lemon juice

Zest from 1 lemon
11 large egg whites at room
   temperature
¼ teaspoon cream of tartar
½ cup granulated sugar
8 large egg yolks

GARNISH

1 tablespoon confectioner's
   sugar

Preheat the oven to 325° F. Grease a nonstick 10-inch tube pan with 2 teaspoons of butter and set aside.

Sift the cornstarch and flour and set aside. Squeeze the lemon juice and set aside. Grate the lemon zest on the fine side of a grater or remove with a citrus zester and chop very fine. Set aside.

In a large mixing bowl, beat the egg whites on high speed with an electric mixer until foamy. Add the cream of tartar and gradually start adding the sugar. Continue beating until the whites hold peaks but are not shiny.

In a food processor fitted with the steel blade or with a whisk or beater, beat the egg yolks with the lemon juice and lemon zest until they are thick and the color has lightened.

Gently fold the flour into the egg whites, then fold in the egg yolks. Gently pour or scoop into the buttered pan. Place the pan in the center of the oven. After 35–40 minutes of baking time, if the top of the cake is browning too quickly, cover loosely with a sheet of aluminum foil. Bake until a skewer inserted in the cake comes out clean (about 1 hour). Remove from the oven and turn onto a cooling rack. Dust with 1 tablespoon of confectioner's sugar before serving.

Variations: The cake can also be served with ½ ounce of freshly chopped or pureed fruit per serving:

Fruit Flavor	Calories per portion
Lemon Spongecake with Strawberries	124
Lemon Spongecake with Raspberries	127
Lemon Spongecake with Blueberries	128
Lemon Spongecake with Pineapple	126
Lemon Spongecake with Peaches	126

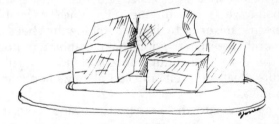

Slimly Scrumptious Cheesecake

Preparation time: about 10 minutes
Baking time: about 20 minutes
Chilling time: 24 hours
Portions: 8
Calories per portion: 182

CRUST

1 teaspoon unsalted butter at
    room temperature
1 tablespoon dry bread crumbs
    (see technique in
    Artichoke Stuffed with
    Ham and Cheese)

¼ teaspoon freshly grated
    nutmeg

FILLING

6 ounces part-skim ricotta cheese at room temperature

10 ounces Neufchâtel cheese at room temperature
4 tablespoons honey
2 large eggs
1 teaspoon vanilla

Butter the bottom and 1 inch up the side of an 8-inch springform or regular round cake pan. Grate the nutmeg and combine in a small bowl with the bread crumbs. Coat the buttered bottom and sides of the pan with the bread crumb–nutmeg mixture. Set aside.

Preheat the oven to 375° F.

Drain the ricotta in a fine sieve. Squeeze the ricotta dry in a cotton or linen towel (see technique in Provençal Vegetable Gratin).

With an electric mixer or by hand, combine the cheeses and beat until very smooth. Blend in the honey and combine thoroughly. In a small bowl, beat the eggs until smooth. Blend gradually with the cheese mixture. Beat very well until completely smooth and creamy. Mix in the vanilla.

Pour the mixture into the prepared pan and bake in the pre-heated oven for 20 minutes. Remove from the oven and cool on a wire rack. When cool, refrigerate the cake, uncovered, for about 24 hours before cutting and eating. Leftover cheesecake can be wrapped in foil or plastic wrap and refrigerated for 1–2 days.

Carob Brownies

Preparation time: about 5 minutes
Baking time: 20 minutes
Portions: 16
Calories per portion: 68

2 ounces unsalted butter
¼ cup honey
¼ cup skim milk
1 ounce carob powder

¾ cup flour (½ whole wheat and ½ all purpose unbleached enriched)
1 ounce walnuts
2 large eggs
½ teaspoon pure vanilla extract

Preheat the oven to 350° F.

Melt the butter and mix in the honey, milk, and carob. Cook for 1–2 minutes, stirring well, until any lumps are dissolved. Set aside to cool slightly.

Combine the flours. Chop the nuts very fine.

In a mixing bowl, beat the eggs. Gradually add the carob mixture, beating well until smooth. Add the flours and mix. Add the nuts and vanilla. Pour into a nonstick 8-inch square baking pan. Place in the oven. Bake until brownies start to leave the sides of the pan and a toothpick inserted in the center comes out clean (about 20 minutes). If brownies start to rise very high in the center, pierce with a skewer or toothpick to deflate.

Transfer the brownies to a wire rack to cool. Cut into 16 squares when cool, then store in an airtight jar or tin.

Pumpkin Bread

Preparation time: about 10 minutes
Baking time: 55–60 minutes
Portions: 20
Calories per portion: 80

2 large eggs
2 tablespoons vegetable oil
2 tablespoons pure maple
   syrup
¾ cup Pumpkin Puree (see
   Index)
½ teaspoon pure vanilla extract

¼ teaspoon cardamom
1 ounce walnuts
¾ cup all-purpose unbleached
   enriched flour
¾ cup whole wheat flour
½ teaspoon baking soda
¼ teaspoon baking powder

Preheat the oven to 350° F. Beat the eggs in a mixing bowl. Add the oil, maple syrup, pumpkin puree, and vanilla, and mix well.

Remove the white, pulpy outer covering of the cardamom seeds with a fingernail or knife. Grind the dark inner seeds with a mortar and pestle or small spice grinder. Chop the nuts very fine and set aside. Combine the flours with the dry ingredients and add to the liquid in the mixing bowl. Mix to combine. Add the nuts and stir.

Pour the batter into an 8½" × 4½" × 2½" nonstick loaf pan. Bake until the loaf is well browned and firm to the touch (55–60 minutes). Remove from the oven. Let the loaf sit for 5 minutes, then turn out onto a cooling rack. Cool for several hours before slicing.

Banana-Nut Bread

The natural sugar in well-ripened bananas is the flavor key to this moist loaf. Keep bananas in a brown paper bag or fruit ripener at room temperature until the skins turn black.

Preparation time: about 10 minutes
Baking time: about 60 minutes
Portions: 20
Calories per portion: 89

2 large eggs
2 tablespoons honey
2 tablespoons vegetable oil
13 ounces ripe bananas
2 tablespoons skim milk
½ teaspoon vanilla

1 ounce walnuts
½ cup all-purpose unbleached enriched flour
¾ cup whole wheat flour
½ teaspoon baking soda
¼ teaspoon baking powder

Preheat the oven to 350° F.

Beat the eggs in a mixing bowl with the honey and oil. Puree the bananas in a food processor fitted with the steel blade or in a blender. Add to the egg mixture and combine. Mix in the milk and vanilla.

Chop the walnuts very fine and set aside. Combine the flours with the other dry ingredients and mix with the banana mixture. Add the chopped nuts. Pour into an 8½" × 4½" × 2½" nonstick loaf pan. Bake until the loaf is well browned and firm to the touch (about 1 hour).

Remove the banana bread from the oven. Let sit 5 minutes on a cooling rack, then turn the loaf out onto the rack to cool for several hours.

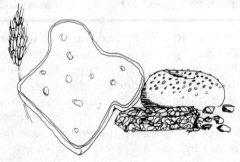

All-American Apple Bread

Preparation time: about 20 minutes
Baking time: 45–50 minutes
Portions: 20
Calories per portion: 70

2 tablespoons unsalted butter
10 ounces Jonathan or
   McIntosh apples
1 teaspoon coriander seeds
1 large egg
2 tablespoons honey

2 tablespoons skim milk
1¾ cups all-purpose
   unbleached enriched flour
½ teaspoon baking powder
½ teaspoon baking soda
¼ teaspoon kosher salt
1 teaspoon vanilla extract

Preheat the oven to 350° F.

Melt the butter in a small pan and set aside.

Peel and core the apples and shred in a food processor or on the coarse side of a vegetable grater. Grind the coriander seeds with a mortar and pestle or a spice grinder. Set aside.

Beat the egg in a mixing bowl. Add the honey, milk, and butter, and mix well. Add the shredded apples and mix. Combine the dry ingredients and add to the apple mixture. Mix well. Add the vanilla and mix. Pour the batter into a nonstick 8½″ × 4½″ × 2½″ loaf pan. Bake until lightly browned and firm to the touch (45–50 minutes).

Transfer from the oven to a cooling rack for 5 minutes. Turn out onto the rack and cool for several hours before slicing.

8
Better-for-You Beverage Snacks

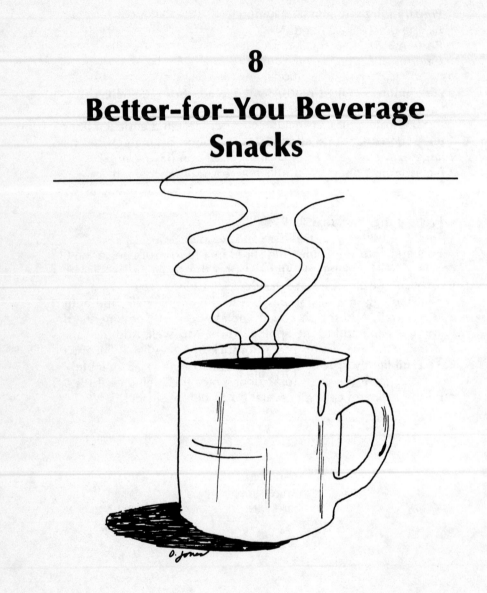

Ever wonder about the success of American soft drinks? The flavors aren't very interesting, and their overpowering sweetness doesn't do much to quench a thirst. Sweetened chemical soft drinks aré a way of life with many Americans and account for a high percentage of our sugar intake. This is one dietary habit that should and can be kicked. Even if you switch to an artificially sweetened soft drink, there is no nutritional advantage. Many of the beverages I offer are not only flavorful and refreshing, but provide some nutrition as well. They make excellent quickly prepared snacks.

Recipes in this chapter include cool and creams fruit shakes, fruit juice spritzers, and spiced hot drinks. Many can easily be transported to the office to combat the temptation of vending machine drinks. Some of the fruit drinks may separate if they are made in advance. No problem—carry them to work in a jar and give them a good shake right before drinking.

If you have access to a refrigerator at work, stock it with small bottles of naturally carbonated or pure seltzer water. Keep a lemon or lime on hand the garnish the drink and you have a pure, natural refresher for less than 1 calorie. That's a better-for-you beverage.

COLD BEVERAGES

Orange Juice Spritzer

Preparation time: about 1 minute
Portions: 1
Calories per portion: 56

**4 ounces freshly squeezed
   orange juice**

**4 ounces naturally sparkling
   water or pure seltzer water**

Combine juice and water and pour over ice in a tall glass. Garnish with a fresh mint leaf or orange slice.

Fruit Juice Spritzers: Prepare with the same proportions as above.

Flavor	Calories per portion
Grapefruit Juice Spritzer	48
Cranberry Juice Spritzer	79
Apple Juice Spritzer	59
Grape Juice Spritzer	84

White Wine Spritzer

This is the drink to order at a cocktail party if you don't want to consume too many empty alcohol calories.

Preparation time: about 30 seconds
Portions: 1
Calories per portion: 75

3 ounces dry white wine
4 ounces naturally sparkling
    water or pure seltzer water

Pour wine and water over ice in a tall glass and mix.

Watermelon Cooler

Preparation time: about 5 minutes
Portions: 1
Calories per portion: 32

4 ounces very ripe watermelon,   **4 ounces naturally sparkling**
    cut into cubes, seeds   **water or pure seltzer water**
    removed   **3 ice cubes**
1 teaspoon lemon juice

GARNISH

Fresh mint leaf or lemon slice

In the food processor fitted with the steel blade or in a blender, shave the ice cubes. Transfer to a tall 12-ounce glass. Puree the watermelon cubes until they are liquid. Add the lemon juice and water and blend. If desired, strain through a sieve to remove any pieces of fiber. Pour into the glass over the shaved ice. Garnish with a mint leaf or lemon slice.

Tomato Juice Cocktail

Preparation time: about 1 minute
Portions: 1
Calories per portion: 41

¾ cup tomato juice
Lemon wedge

Freshly ground black pepper
Dash of angostura bitters

Pour tomato juice into a glass and squeeze lemon over it. Drop lemon wedge into juice. Grind black pepper over the top and add a dash of bitters. Mix well. Add 2–3 ice cubes and drink right away.

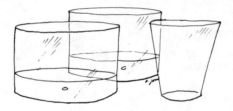

Banana Bonanza

Preparation time: about 2 minutes
Portions: 1
Calories per portion: 96

1 4-ounce very ripe banana
⅓ cup skim milk
Freshly grated nutmeg

Peel the banana and cut into chunks. In the blender or a food processor fitted with the steel blade, puree the banana. Add the milk and combine. Pour into a tall glass and dust the top with freshly grated nutmeg.

O.J. Shake

Preparation time: about 3 minutes
Portions: 1
Calories per portion: 96

⅓ **cup freshly squeezed orange**   ⅔ **cup skim milk**
     juice   **1 ice cube (1″ × 1″ × ¾″)**

Process ingredients in a blender or in a food processor fitted with the steel blade until frothy and thick (about 50 seconds). Drink right away.

Tart Apple Tempter

Preparation time: about 2 minutes
Portions: 1
Calories per portion: 73

1 tablespoon lemon juice   **4 ounces naturally sparkling**
4 ounces apple juice   **water or pure seltzer water**
½ **teaspoon honey**

GARNISH

Fresh mint leaf or lemon slice

In a tall glass, stir the lemon juice, apple juice, and honey until the honey dissolves. Add the water. Fill the glass with ice and garnish with a fresh mint leaf or lemon slice.

Apple Delight

Preparation time: about 1 minute
Portions: 1
Calories per portion: 69

⅓ **cup apple juice**
⅓ **cup skim milk**

1 ice cube (1″ × 1″ × ¾″)
Freshly grated cinnamon

Combine the apple juice and milk in a blender or food processor fitted with the steel blade. With the machine running, add the ice cube through the feed tube. (If using blender, check manufacturer's guidelines for chopping ice.) Process for about 30 seconds until the mixture is thick and frothy. Pour into a 14-ounce glass or mug and garnish with freshly grated cinnamon. Drink right away.

Pineapple Supreme

Preparation time: about 2 minutes
Portions: 1
Calories per portion: 110

3 ounces fresh pineapple
   chunks
¾ **cup skim milk**

Process the pineapple in a blender or the bowl of a food processor fitted with the steel blade until the pineapple is finely chopped. Add the milk to the bowl and process until thick and frothy (about 60 seconds). Pour into a 14-ounce glass or mug. Drink right away.

Tangy Cantaloupe Quencher

Preparation time: about 3 minutes
Portions: 1
Calories per portion: 107

6 ounces cleaned cantaloupe
½ **cup skim milk**
2 tablespoons Slim Snacks
   Yogurt (see Index)

Freshly grated nutmeg or
   cinnamon

Cut the cantaloupe into chunks. Place in a blender or in a food processor fitted with the steel blade. Puree. Add the milk and the yogurt and blend until just incorporated. Pour into a tall glass and dust with freshly grated nutmeg or cinnamon.

Thick 'n' Rich Carob Shake

Preparation time: about 5 minutes
Cooling time: 30 minutes
Portions: 2
Calories per portion: 51

1 tablespoon carob powder   **¾ cup skim milk**
1 teaspoon honey   **3 ice cubes (1″ × 1″ × ¾″)**

Combine the carob and honey in a saucepan. Add the milk and stir well. Heat until the milk is hot and the carob powder is dissolved. Cool.

Put the carob milk in a food processor fitted with the steel blade or in a blender. With the machine running, add 3 ice cubes, one at a time, through the feed tube.

Process until thick and foamy. Pour into 2 tall glasses and drink right away.

Mocha Shake

Preparation time: about 5 minutes
Cooling time: 30 minutes
Portions: 2
Calories per portion: 40

1 tablespoon carob powder   **¼ cup strong brewed coffee**
1 teaspoon honey   **(French roast or espresso)**
                                       ½ cup skim milk

Prepare according to the directions in the preceding recipe, adding the coffee to the milk when heating it with the carob powder and honey.

HOT BEVERAGES

Mint Tea

This recipe provides a most refreshing change from regular tea. Grow a profusion of mint in your summer herb garden and you'll have plenty to dry for soothing, caffeine-free mint tea all winter long.

Preparation time: about 5 minutes
Portions: 1
Calories per portion: 8

**3 tablespoons tightly packed
   dry mint leaves or 6
   tablespoons tightly packed
   fresh mint leaves (to taste;
   different mints vary in
   strength)
8 ounces hot water**

Place the leaves in a ceramic teapot, either loose or in a tea ball. Pour hot water over. Cover with the lid and steep for 5 minutes. Pour and drink. Garnish with thin lemon slice if desired.

Iced Mint Tea: Prepare as above. When tea is steeped, pour into a cup or glass and cool to room temperature. Pour into a tall glass filled with ice and garnish with a fresh mint leaf or lemon slice.

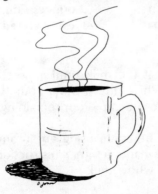

Hot Carob Drink

Preparation time: about 3 minutes
Portions: 1
Calories per portion: 128

1 tablespoon carob powder
1 teaspoon honey
¼ cup water

1 cup skim milk
½ teaspoon pure vanilla extract

In a small saucepan, combine the carob powder, honey, water, and milk. Stir well, then cook over medium heat until the mixture becomes hot. Stir constantly. As the milk heats, use a wire whisk, rotary beater, or electric beater to whip it to a froth. When the milk is hot and frothy, add the vanilla and drink right away.

Light Cappuccino

Preparation time: about 3 minutes
Portions: 1
Calories per portion: 26

6 ounces freshly brewed
espresso or dark roast
coffee

2 ounces skim milk
Freshly grated cinnamon

Brew the coffee. Heat the milk until almost boiling, then pour into a shallow bowl. Whisk until frothy. Pour the milk and coffee simultaneously into a coffee cup. Pour remaining froth on top. Dust with grated cinnamon.

(This drink can also be made using an automatic espresso/cappuccino maker. Follow manufacturer's instructions, substituting the skim milk for cream or whole milk.)

Mulled Cider

Preparation time: about 7 minutes
Portions: 1
Calories per portion: 111

6 ounces apple juice or cider
1-inch-long piece of cinnamon
   stick

1 slice of lemon
1 teaspoon honey

Combine all the ingredients except the honey in a nonaluminum saucepan. Heat gently until almost boiling, then remove from the heat and cover. Steep for 5 minutes. Stir in honey and drink right away.

Hot Spiced Wine

Preparation time: about 7 minutes
Portions: 2
Calories per portion: 94

7 ounces dry red wine
1 slice lemon
1-inch-long piece of cinnamon
   stick

1 clove
½ teaspoon honey

Combine all the ingredients except the honey in a nonaluminum saucepan. Heat gently. Cover and steep, off the heat, for 5 minutes. Stir in the honey and pour into mugs. Drink right away.

9
Postscript on Crunch Cravings

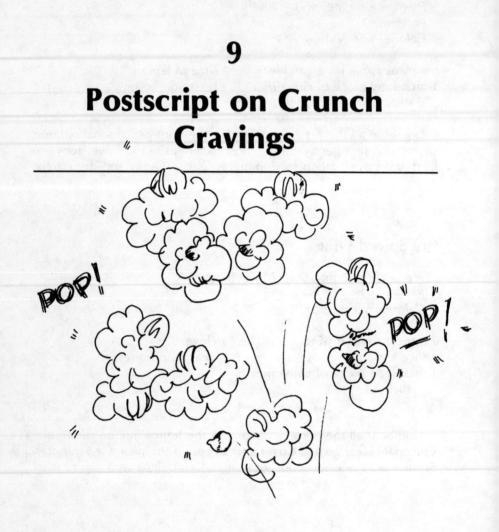

This chapter is a postscript for crunchaholics. If you have tried some of the recipes in the preceding chapters, you are now starting to realize what a wealth of alternatives there are to traditional snack foods.

It is only for the hard-core crunchaholics, those who aren't truly satisfied without something exploding inside their mouths, that I have included this short list of suggestions. They are better options for someone who craves crunch than are high-fat, high-sugar, high-salt processed snack foods.

It is my hope that, as you discover the real taste satisfaction of the fresh foods in slim-snacks recipes, you will need to turn to this chapter less and less.

Fresh Bean Sprouts

Sprouting time: 5–6 days
Yield: 5 ounces

**¾ ounce sprouting beans (a
  mixture of beans or all
  mung beans, available in
  health food stores, bulk
  food stores, and some
  supermarkets)**

In a 1-quart wide-mouth glass jar, place the beans. Fill the jar three-quarters full with warm water. Cover the mouth of the jar with a double thickness of cheesecloth and secure tightly with a rubber band or the metal ring if using a Mason jar. Shake the seeds in the water and drain off the water. Lay the jar on its side.

Repeat the above procedure every morning and evening until the seeds are fully sprouted (5–6 days). When the beans are sprouted, store in the refrigerator for 3–4 days. Use in recipes or as Munch-a-Sprout snack.

Munch-a-Sprout

Preparation time: none, if sprouts are already sprouted
Portions: 1
Calories per portion: 20

2 ounces sprouts

When you feel the urge for some mindless munching, reach into the refrigerator for some sprouts.

Toasted Soy Nuts

Preparation time: about 5 minutes
Soaking time: at least 12 hours
Toasting time: about 40 minutes
Portions: 9
Calories per portion: 80

**6¼ ounces dry yellow soy
    beans (available in health
    food and bulk food stores)**

Soak the soy beans in 3–4 cups cold water for at least 12 hours. Drain and rinse well. Drain again.

Spread the beans on a towel and blot dry with another towel.

Preheat the oven to 350° F.

Place the beans on a large baking sheet so they are in a single layer. Place in the oven and toast for about 40 minutes. Shake the beans or stir them several times during the toasting so they brown evenly. They are done when they are golden-brown and parched-looking. Remove from the oven and sprinkle lightly with salt, if desired. Cool and store in an airtight container in a cool place. These will keep for several weeks.

Variations: Sprinkle the soy nuts lightly with curry powder, paprika, or chili powder after toasting.

Flaked Whole-Grain Cereals

Flaked whole-grain or puffed cereals are a better bet for snacking than junk crunchies, which are extremely high in fat, sugar, and salt.

Portions: a 1-ounce portion of wheat, corn, rye, or barley whole-grain flaked cereal
Calories per portion: 110

Puffed Cereals

Portions: a ½-ounce portion of puffed wheat or puffed rice cereal
Calories per portion: 50

Toasted Pita Wedges

These crisp wedges make a great low-fat and low-calorie party dipper.

Preparation time: about 5 minutes
Portions: 8
Calories per portion: 18

1 whole pita bread (see Index)

Preheat the oven to 350° F.
Cut the pita round into 8 equal wedges. Place the wedges on a baking sheet and bake for 5 minutes or until very crisp. Remove and eat hot or cold. The toasted wedges can be stored for up to a week in an airtight container.

Parmesan Popcorn

Preparation time: about 5 minutes
Portions: 1
Calories per portion: 37

**1 teaspoon grated imported
   Parmesan cheese, very
   loosely packed
1 cup plain popcorn, popped**

Grate the cheese and set aside. Pop the corn in a hot-air popper according to the manufacturer's instructions. Remove 1 cup of the popped corn and toss in a bowl with the Parmesan.

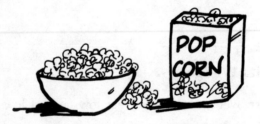

Currycorn

Preparation time: about 5 minutes
Portions: 1
Calories per portion: 30

**1 cup plain popcorn, popped
Curry powder**

Pop the corn in a hot-air popper according to the manufacturer's instructions. Place 1 cup of the corn in a bowl and sprinkle lightly with curry powder. Toss and sprinkle again so that all the popcorn is coated lightly.

Papricorn

Preparation time: about 5 minutes
Portions: 1
Calories per portion: 30

1 cup plain popcorn, popped
Imported paprika

Pop the corn in a hot-air popper according to the manufacturer's instructions. Place 1 cup of the corn in a bowl and sprinkle lightly with paprika. Toss the corn and sprinkle lightly again.

Oven Potato Chips

Preparation time: about 3 minutes
Soaking time: several hours
Baking time: about 20 minutes
Portions: 50 chips
Calories per portion: 4

1 10-ounce baking potato, of
    uniform width
Cold water

Scrub the potato but do not peel. On a vegetable slicer or with a food processor slicing disc, slice the potato into $\frac{1}{8}$-inch-thick slices. (It is important that the slices are a uniform thickness for even baking.) Place the slices in a large bowl of cold water and let sit for at least 2 hours or as long as 5–6 hours.

Preheat the oven to 400° F.

Rinse the potatoes well under cold running water. Place the slices on 2 baking sheets (with at least $\frac{1}{2}$ inch of space between each slice). Bake until the chips are nicely browned (about 20 minutes). Remove from the oven and remove gently with a spatula or pancake turner. Sprinkle with salt if desired. Chips are best when hot and crisp. They can be left at room temperature for several hours, then recrisped for a few minutes in the oven.

Roasted Squash or Pumpkin Seeds

Preparation time: about 5 minutes
Drying time: 1 hour
Roasting time: about 10 minutes
1 snack portion: ½ ounce seeds
Calories per portion: 79

**1 ounce seeds from Spaghetti
    Squash Parmesan (see
    Index)**

**2 ounces seeds from Pumpkin
    Puree (see Index)**

Pick the seeds from the pulp and rinse quickly under cold water.
Spread the seeds on a towel and pat dry with another towel. Place
the seeds on a fresh towel and let dry for 1 hour.

Preheat the oven to 350° F. Spread the seeds on a baking sheet
and place in the oven. Bake for 10 minutes or until golden brown.
Remove immediately and place in a bowl. Sprinkle lightly with salt,
if desired. The seeds will keep for weeks in a cool, dry spot.

Index